Color Atlas of Preoperative Staging and Surgical Treatment Options in Rectal Cancer

Color Atlas of Preoperative Staging and Surgical Treatment Options in Rectal Cancer

Tomas M. Heimann, M.D., F.A.C.S.
Professor of Surgery
Mount Sinai School of Medicine
New York, New York
Attending Surgeon
Mount Sinai Hospital
New York, New York

Arnold H. Szporn, M.D.
Assistant Professor of Pathology
Mount Sinai School of Medicine
New York, New York
Assistant Attending Pathologist
Mount Sinai Hospital
New York, New York

Williams & Wilkins

A WAVERLY COMPANY

BALTIMORE • PHILADELPHIA • LONDON • PARIS • BANGKOK
BUENOS AIRES • HONG KONG • MUNICH • SYDNEY • TOKYO • WROCLAW

Editor: Johnathan W. Pine, Jr
Production Coordinator: Dana M. Soares
Typesetter: Better Graphics, Inc.
Printer: Quebecar Printing Book Group

351 West Camden Street
Baltimore, Maryland 21201-2436 USA

Rose Tree Corporate Center
1400 North Providence Road
Building II, Suite 5025
Media, Pennsylvania 19063-2043 USA

Accurate indications, adverse reactions and dosage schedules for drugs are provided in this book, but it is possible that they may change. The reader is urged to review the package information data of the manufacturers of the medications mentioned.

Printed in the United States of America

First Edition

ISBN: 0-683-30341-4

The publishers have made every effort to trace the copyright holders for borrowed material. If they have inadvertently overlooked any, they will be pleased to make the necessary arrangements at the first opportunity.

To purchase additional copies of this book, call our customer service department at **(800) 638-0672** or fax orders to **(800) 447-8438**. For other book services, including chapter reprints and large quantity sales, ask for the Special Sales department.

Canadian customers should call **(800) 665-1148**, or fax **(800) 665-0103**. For all other calls originating outside of the United States, please call **(410) 528-4223** or fax us at **(410) 528-8550**.

Visit Williams & Wilkins on the Internet: http://www.wwilkins.com or contact our customer service department at **custserv@wwilkins.com**. Williams & Wilkins customer service representatives are available from 8:30 am to 6:00 pm, EST, Monday through Friday, for telephone access.

98 99 00
1 2 3 4 5 6 7 8 9 10

Dedication

To Wendy, David, and Gabrielle.
To Rachel and Joshua.

Acknowledgment

The authors would like to thank the Hildegarde D. Becher Foundation, Inc. for their generous support of this project.

Contents

Chapter 1

Preoperative Staging of Rectal Cancer

The ability to accurately stage rectal cancer prior to surgical excision significantly improves the surgical and adjuvant treatment options. The accessibility of these tumors to visual inspection and digital palpation allows a limited degree of evaluation prior to decision as to appropriate treatment. Large fixed lesions that appear locally advanced, for example, are often treated with preoperative radiation, and if necessary, with a complementary colostomy. Small villous tumors, on the other hand, are less likely to have a malignant component and are often treated with local excision thereby avoiding a colostomy.

Early attempts at preoperative staging were crude and lacked the accuracy needed to reliably determine depth of invasion and presence of nodal metastasis. The advent of computerized axial tomography has improved our ability to determine the extent of the tumor but it does not provide sufficient definition of the tissue layers to accurately stage early lesions. Nodal metastasis may be suspected on computerized tomography, but the lymph nodes must be large and there is no distinction between hyperplastic and metastatic nodes. Computerized tomography is most useful in evaluation of locally advanced lesions and distant metastasis.

Endorectal sonography provides detailed examination of the tumor, its location, size, depth of invasion, and presence of nodal metastasis. Although various systems are available, we have used a rigid probe with a 360° rotating lateral viewing transducer at the tip (Bruel and Kjaer). This system operates at a frequency of 7 or 10 MHz and produces axial sections of the rectum with excellent definition of the bowel wall, tumor, and adjacent structures. The 10-MHz probe provides improved resolution of the layers of the bowel wall but the higher frequency also results in a shorter focal length.

We currently use endorectal sonography as part of the initial evaluation of most patients with rectal cancer. Patient preparation consists of an enema 2 hr prior to the office visit. Following a history and physical exam, the patient is positioned in the modified jackknife position on a proctology examination table. A digital exam is performed to determine whether the tumor is palpable, its location, mobility, consistency, and distance from the anal verge. A rigid sigmoidoscopy is then performed and the distance of the tumor from the anal verge, its size, appearance, and location are recorded. The endorectal ultrasound probe is then introduced into the rectum and advanced proximal to the tumor. The balloon surrounding the ultrasound crystal is inflated with 60 cc of water and the probe is gradually withdrawn as the examination is performed. After an initial exam, it is often useful to deflate the balloon, advance the probe proximal to the tumor again and repeat the study in order to obtain the best representative sections which are then printed for a permanent record.

The entire rectum is accessible to this probe but, in our experience, proximal lesions are more difficult to study. The focal range of the 7-MHz probe is 2 to 4.5 cm with a focal length of 3 cm. The difference in tissue density of the rectal wall produces a five-layer pattern which is used to determine tumor stage. These layers are usually best seen with the transducer in the center of the rectal lumen. The inner hyperechoic (white) layer is the balloon–mucosa interface, the next hypoechoic layer (dark) represents the muscularis mucosa, then the hyperechoic submucosal interface is seen, followed by the hypoechoic muscularis propria, and finally the hyperechoic perirectal fat interface forms the outer layer. These layers are interrupted and distorted when invaded by tumor.

Rectal tumors are hypoechoic. Tumor invasion disrupts the hyperechoic layers and widens the hypoechoic layers. Disruption of the hyperechoic layers (submucosa and perirectal fat) provides a very precise indication of tumor invasion with a predictive value of over 95%. Prediction of invasion of the muscularis propria is somewhat less accurate (85%) since both the tumor and the muscularis are hypoechoic. Minimal amount of thickening of the muscularis propria is more difficult to detect than disruption of a contrasting hyperechoic layer. Failure to diagnose thickening due to tumor invasion is a common cause of understaging of the tumor. Overstaging occurs when surrounding inflammation obscures the hyperechoic layers simulating tumor invasion. Understaging may also occur when the tumor produces narrowing and angulation of the lumen and does not allow passage of the probe. Although the distal portion of the tumor is seen, the depth of invasion at this level may be more superficial than in the central portion of the tumor. Enlarged lymph nodes may also be missed since they are often located adjacent or proximal to the tumor (see Tables 1.1 and 1.2).

Normal lymph nodes are usually not visible on sonography. Enlarged lymph nodes, when present, are often found at the same level as the tumor or just proximal to it. It is unusual to find metastatic nodes located distal to the tumor. Patients without visible nodes have a low possibility of having nodal metastasis (14%). Small lymph nodes less than 5 mm in diameter have less than 20% chance of containing metastatic disease. Lymph nodes between 5 and 9 mm have a 45% probability of metastasis, and larger nodes have a 70% chance of containing tumor metastasis. Hypoechoic areas and irregular borders increase the possibility of nodal metastasis. The accuracy of endorectal

TABLE 1.1 Histologic Tumor Classification

PRIMARY TUMOR
T1:   Tumor invading submucosa
T2:   Tumor invading muscularis propria
T3:   Tumor invading perirectal fat
T4:   Tumor invading adjacent structures

REGIONAL LYMPH NODES
N0:   No regional lymph node metastasis
N1:   Perirectal lymph node metastasis

TYPE OF CLASSIFICATION
U: Ultrasound staging
P: Histologic staging

TABLE 1.2 Modified Dukes Classification

DUKES A:	Tumor invading the submucosa
DUKES B1:	Tumor invading muscularis propria
DUKES B2:	Tumor invading perirectal fat
DUKES C1:	Tumor invading muscularis propria with lymph node metastasis
DUKES C2:	Tumor invading perirectal fat with lymph node metastasis
DUKES D:	Presence of distant metastasis

sonography in predicting nodal involvement has been reported as ranging from 80 to 88%. Attempts have also been made to obtain biopsies of perirectal nodes using a transrectal sonographically guided, 18-gauge, spring-loaded biopsy needle. Lymphoid tissue was obtained in 69% of the patients in whom a biopsy was attempted and a histologic diagnosis of metastatic carcinoma was made in 50%.

SURGICAL TREATMENT OF DISTAL RECTAL CANCER

The surgical procedures described in this *Atlas* range from local excision to extended abdominoperineal resection with intraoperative brachytherapy. Patients with villous adenomas and those presenting with small carcinomas invading the submucosa or superficial muscularis propria without sonographic evidence of nodal metastasis are often treated with local excision. This choice is especially important in distal lesions that otherwise require abdominoperineal resection. We prefer local excision to fulguration or destruction with radiotherapy since with local excision, the margins and the depth of invasion may be carefully examined. Only well-differentiated small tumors less than 3 cm in diameter which are superficially invasive are good candidates for local excision. Presence of enlarged lymph nodes on sonography should be a contraindication to local excision. Lesions near the dentate line amenable to local excision are best treated by transanal excision, whereas more proximal lesions are approached using a posterior proctotomy with excision of the coccyx. Regardless of the approach used, the tumor should be excised in one piece, with 1-cm margins using full-thickness excision. The tumor should be pinned and oriented on a flat surface and the margins inked for histologic examination. Fifteen percent of patients with superficial invasion of the muscularis propria have nodal metastasis. It is interesting to note that the actuarial 5-yr survival for patients with rectal cancer treated by local excision before the advent of endorectal sonography is 86%. Since incomplete local excision is usually detected on histologic exam, treatment failures most likely represent patients with nodal metastasis. Endorectal sonography should help identify patients with nodal metastasis thereby improving selection for local excision.

More advanced distal rectal tumors are treated with low anterior resection and either stapled distal rectal anastomosis or hand-sewn coloanal anastomosis. We often use an everted double stapled technique for small distal rectal cancers and extensive villous adenomas. This technique consists of mobilization of the rectum to level of the levator muscles with eversion of the rectum and the tumor through the anal canal. The rectum is then transected from the perineal side with a stapler and the remaining segment of anorectum is then replaced into the perineum. An end-to-end anastomosis (EEA) stapler is then used to restore intestinal continuity. This technique allows for perineal transection of the distal rectum under direct vision and the distal margin of the tumor is clearly visible. The functional results with this technique are superior to those seen with hand-sewn coloanal anastomosis.

Proctectomy with mucosectomy and hand-sewn coloanal anastomosis is useful in cases where the tumor is close to the dentate line and would otherwise require an abdominoperineal resection. In general, we prefer to perform the resection first and use adjuvant chemoradiation, if needed, following healing of the coloanal anastomosis. Patients with extensive tumor and those with multiple enlarged nodes on sonography undergo preoperative chemoradiation. In cases where there is regression after chemoradiation it may become possible to perform a coloanal anastomosis. If there is significant residual tumor on endorectal sonography after chemoradiation is completed, we have used abdominoperineal resection with intraoperative brachytherapy. We are reluctant to perform coloanal anastomosis in patients with a high local recurrence potential since the functional results deteriorate very rapidly after development of recurrent disease.

OTHER APPLICATIONS OF ENDORECTAL SONOGRAPHY

Endosonography is also very useful for studying anal lesions and sphincteric problems. Anal studies are performed using a water-filled plastic cap instead of the balloon. The sphincteric muscles are well seen and sonography is very useful in the evaluation of patients who develop fecal incontinence following surgical procedures and obstetric trauma. Anorectal sonographic studies using hydrogen peroxide enhancement have been used to define the location of complex fistulas in patients with inflammatory bowel disease and recurrent anal fistulas.

Endorectal sonography is also used to monitor the results of chemoradiation in patients with squamous cell anal cancer. Pretreatment sonographic staging is compared to post-treatment studies and subsequent follow-up. Patients with advanced rectal cancer receiving preoperative chemoradiation are also often followed with serial endorectal sonography. It is important to note, however, that radiation produces scarring and edema of the rectal wall and adjacent structures making postradiation staging less accurate. Nevertheless, comparison with pretreatment studies may show clear tumor regression and even disappearance of previously present enlarged lymph nodes.

Patients with rectal cancer have a significant possibility of developing local recurrence. Follow-up of patients following rectal resection is improved with the addition of endorectal sonography. Initial evaluation of the anastomosis is important since postsurgical changes may be misinterpreted as possible recurrent disease. Serial evaluations and correlation with carcinoembryonic antigen (CEA) levels and endoscopic findings are necessary to confirm the presence of local recurrence. Early diagnosis may allow for a curative secondary resection with coloanal anastomosis or abdominoperineal resection before the onset of distant metastasis.

The following pages present detailed descriptions and illustrations of patients with anorectal tumors and sphincteric injury which have been referred to us for evaluation and treatment. The format used describes presenting symptoms, physical examination, endorectal sonographic findings, surgical treatment, and tumor grade and stage. Cases that were over or understaged are described with the accompanying histologic correlation and an explanation for the resulting inaccurate sonographic stage. Several patients with advanced tumors treated with preoperative chemoradiation are also presented to demonstrate the usefulness of endorectal sonography in assessing the response of the tumor to neoadjuvant treatment.

Sonographic studies in several areas of medicine are becoming part of the initial evaluation of the patient. Endosonography in a patient with rectal cancer is an important extension of the physical exam. The treatment of rectal cancer is difficult and better decisions are made when tumor stage is known before surgical excision is performed. Pretreatment sonographic staging is most effective when the information is used to plan further course of treatment.

SELECTED READINGS

Adams WJ, Wong WD: Endorectal ultrasonic detection of malignancy within rectal villous lesions. *Dis Colon Rectum* 38:1093–1096, 1995.

Bernini A, Deen KI, Maddoff RD, et al: Preoperative adjuvant radiation with chemotherapy for rectal cancer: its impact on stage of the disease and the role of endorectal ultrasound. *Ann Surg Oncol* 3:131–135, 1996.

Cheong DMO, Nogueras JJ, Wexner SD, et al: Anal endosonography for recurrent anal fistulas: image enhancement with hydrogen peroxide. *Dis Colon Rectum* 36:1158–1160, 1993.

Falk PM, Blatchford GJ, Cali RL, et al: Transanal ultrasound and manometry in the evaluation of fecal incontinence. *Dis Colon Rectum* 37:468–472, 1994.

Felt-Bersma RJF, van Baren R, Koorevaar M, et al: Unsuspected sphincter defects shown by anal endosonography after anorectal surgery. *Dis Colon Rectum* 38:249–253, 1995.

Fleshman JW, Myerson RJ, Fry RD, et al: Accuracy of transrectal ultrasound in predicting pathologic stage of rectal cancer before and after preoperative radiation therapy. *Dis Colon Rectum* 35:823–829, 1992.

Katsura Y, Yamada K, Ishizawa T, et al: Endorectal ultrasonography for the assessment of wall invasion and lymph node metastasis in rectal cancer. *Dis Colon Rectum* 35:362–368, 1992.

Meade PW, Blatchford GJ, Thornson AG, et al: Preoperative chemoradiation downstages locally advanced ultrasound-staged rectal cancer. *Am J Surg* 170:609–613, 1995.

Milsom JW, Czyrko C, Hull TL, et al: Preoperative biopsy of pararectal lymph nodes in rectal cancer using endoluminal ultrasonography. *Dis Colon Rectum* 37:364–368, 1994.

Sentovich SM, Blatchford GJ, Falk PM, et al: Transrectal ultrasound of rectal tumors. *Am J Surg* 166:638–641, 1993.

Solomon MJ, Mcleod RS: Endoluminal transrectal ultrasonography: accuracy, reliability, validity. *Dis Colon Rectum* 36:200–205, 1993.

Williamson PR, Hellinger MD, Larach SW, et al: Endorectal ultrasound of T3 and T4 rectal cancers after preoperative chemoradiation. *Dis Colon Rectum* 39:45–49, 1996.

Chapter 2
Anatomic Considerations

Anatomic Considerations

Nearly all of the sonographic pictures used in this atlas were obtained with a Bruel and Kjaer system using a standard 7- or 10-MHz endorectal probe. This probe may be used with a plastic cap for sphincter studies or with a balloon for rectal imaging. A Sony thermal printer was used to obtain copies of selected images. This system is relatively simple to use and provides good quality images at a reasonable cost. We examine the patient on a proctology table in the modified jackknife position. Following external inspection and digital exam, rigid sigmoidoscopy is performed to determine the location of the lesion and its distance from the anal verge. The sigmoidoscope is then removed and endorectal sonography is performed. In patients with rectal cancer, the probe is advanced proximal to the tumor before the balloon is inflated with about 60 cc of water. As the probe is gradually withdrawn, serial images are obtained.

We use endosonography most often for preoperative staging of rectal cancer. It is also used for postoperative follow-up and sphincter studies. We find that endorectal sonography is most useful for distal rectal tumors. Lesions located above 14 cm from the anal verge are more difficult to study with the rigid probe. This also applies to advanced circumferential lesions and tumors producing severe angulation of the lumen. In any situation where the probe cannot be freely advanced proximal to the tumor, the depth of invasion and the presence of nodal metastasis is difficult to ascertain.

TYPES OF PROBES

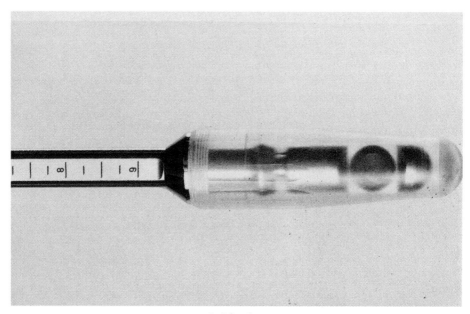

Sphincter
Fig. 2.1

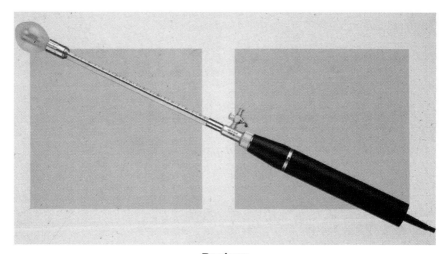

Rectum
Fig. 2.2

Figures 2.1 and 2.2 show the types of probes used for endorectal sonography. The probe above has a rigid plastic cap which is filled with water and is used for sphincteric studies. The probe on the bottom has a water-filled balloon covering the ultrasound crystal and is designed for evaluation of rectal lesions. The crystal rotates during the examination and provides a cross-sectional view of the rectal wall and adjacent structures. Even though the patient is in the prone jackknife position during the study, all sonographic images in this atlas are oriented so the anterior wall is superior and the left side of the image represents the right side of the patient. This provides a cross-sectional image that is oriented in the same fashion as the images seen on a conventional computed tomography (CT) scan.

ANAL SPHINCTER

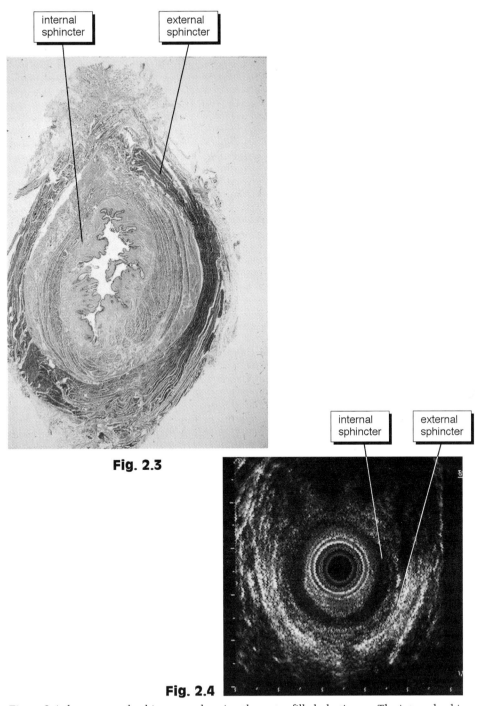

internal sphincter

external sphincter

Fig. 2.3

internal sphincter

external sphincter

Fig. 2.4

Figure 2.4 shows an anal sphincter study using the water-filled plastic cap. The internal sphincter is visible as a hypoechoic circular layer around the hyperechoic mucosal interface. Surrounding the internal sphincter is a layer of mixed echogenicity which represents the external sphincter. The anatomic cross section taken at the level of the sphincter muscles (Fig. 2.3) provides a detailed view of the actual layers corresponding to those seen in the sonogram. This sonographic system provides precise anatomic detail of the sphincters and is very useful in the study of sphincteric injuries in patients with continence problems.

FEMALE RECTAL SONOGRAPHY

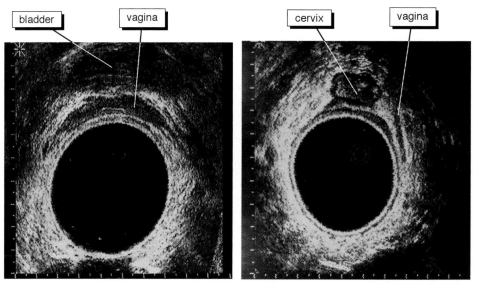

bladder | vagina

cervix | vagina

Fig. 2.5   Fig. 2.6

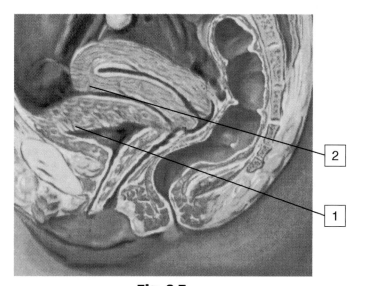

2

1

Fig. 2.7

Sonographic sections through the distal and mid rectum in a female patient using a water-filled balloon around the ultrasound transducer (Fig. 2.7). The image on the left shows a cross section of the rectum showing the vagina anteriorly and the bladder in front of the vagina (Fig. 2.5). The image on the right side shows the cervix, and part of the vagina anterior to the rectum (Fig. 2.6). This sonographic system is designed to provide information about the layers of the rectal wall and the surrounding lymph nodes. The adjacent organs are usually well seen and are used as anatomic reference points to determine the location of the tumor.

10

MALE RECTAL SONOGRAPHY

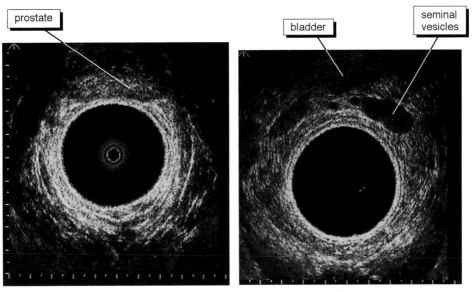

Fig. 2.8   Fig. 2.9

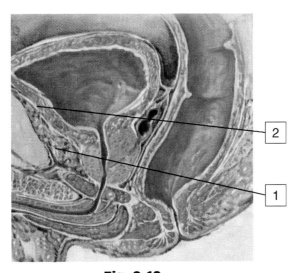

Fig. 2.10

Sonographic view of the rectum in a male patient. As seen on the anatomic section (Fig. 2.10), the image on the left is at the level of the prostate (Fig. 2.8). The one on the right is more proximal and shows the rectum at the level of the seminal vesicles (Fig. 2.9). The bladder is seen anterior to the seminal vesicles. These landmarks are helpful in determining the structures adjacent to the tumor. The exact level of the tumor and especially the distance from the anal verge is best measured during rigid sigmoidoscopy with the patient in the prone jackknife position. These measurements are especially important in low rectal lesions where a decision needs to be made whether sphincter preservation is possible.

Chapter 3
Sphincteric Studies

Sphincteric Studies

Sphincteric studies using the water-filled plastic cap allow for precise evaluation of anatomic injury occurring as a result of previous surgery or other trauma. The presence of disruption of the sphincter muscles is clearly seen and the images can be correlated with manometric findings. Sphincteric studies are also useful in delineating the location of fistulas, especially when they are enhanced by injection of hydrogen peroxide. Sonography of the anal canal is also used to stage anal squamous carcinomas prior to therapy with chemoradiation.

HEMORROIDECTOMY

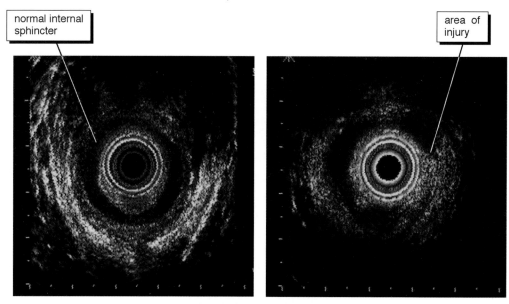

normal internal sphincter

area of injury

SPHINCTERIC INJURY

Fig. 3.1   **Fig. 3.2**

CLINICAL PRESENTATION

43-yr-old woman who developed fecal incontinence following hemorrhoidectomy and sphincterotomy 1 yr ago.

PHYSICAL EXAM

INSPECTION: No abnormalities seen.

DIGITAL EXAM: No stricture palpable, slightly decreased resting sphincter tone with markedly decreased squeeze tone. Area of weakness palpable in left posterolateral side.

SIGMOIDOSCOPY: Normal rectal mucosa.

ENDORECTAL SONOGRAPHY

Figure 3.2 shows hypertrophy of the internal sphincter muscle with scarring of the left posterolateral portion due to surgical injury. The area of scarring occupies nearly one-quarter of the circumference and is hyperechoic. The portion of internal sphincter muscle that is intact is hypoechoic and retracted. The right posterior and anterior segments of the internal sphincter also appear thinned out and may represent the site of additional hemorrhoidectomy with partial muscle damage. The figure on the left (Fig. 3.1) represents a normal section taken at about the same level in a different patient.

TRAUMATIC DELIVERY

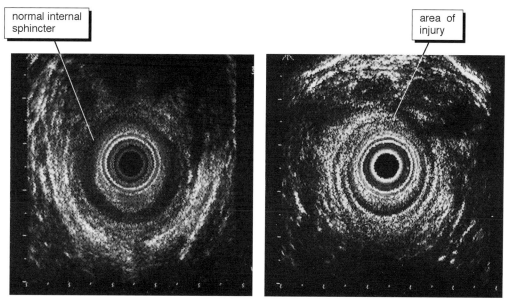

normal internal sphincter

area of injury

SPHINCTERIC INJURY

Fig. 3.3   **Fig. 3.4**

CLINICAL PRESENTATION

30-yr-old woman who developed fecal incontinence following traumatic delivery resulting in a rectovaginal tear. The patient remains incontinent after two operations to repair the sphincter muscles. There is no evidence of a rectovaginal fistula.

PHYSICAL EXAM

INSPECTION: Anterior scarring, no rectovaginal fistula seen.
DIGITAL EXAM: Severely decreased resting and squeeze sphincter tone.
SIGMOIDOSCOPY: Normal rectal mucosa.

ENDORECTAL SONOGRAPHY

Figure 3.4 shows injury to anterior portion of the internal and external sphincter muscles with retraction and replacement by scar tissue. The residual normal sphincter muscles are seen in the posterolateral area. The normal internal sphincter is hypoechoic and the normal external sphincter is hyperechoic and surrounds the internal sphincter. The scar tissue occupies the entire anterior portion and obscures the normal anatomy. The scarred area appears to have mixed echogenicity and the various anatomic layers are blended together. Figure 3.3 represents a normal study for comparison.

ANAL SQUAMOUS CELL CARCINOMA

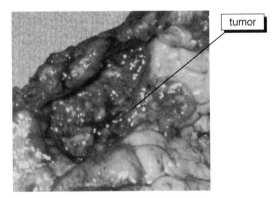

Fig. 3.5

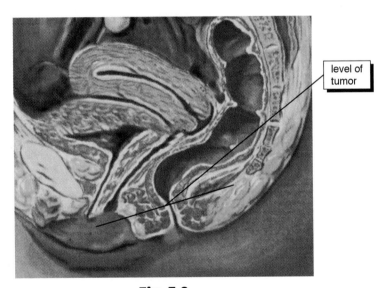

Fig. 3.6

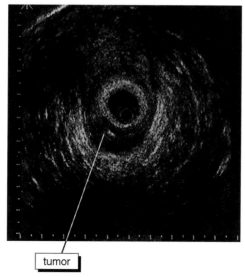

tumor

Fig. 3.7

CLINICAL PRESENTATION

43-yr-old woman presenting with rectal bleeding for 5 months and more recently increased anal pressure and straining during bowel movements.

PHYSICAL EXAM

INSPECTION: Flat ulcerated posterior anal lesion extending to the dentate line. (Figs. 3.5 and 3.6)

DIGITAL EXAM: Hard ulcerated anal lesion 3 × 2 cm in size.

SIGMOIDOSCOPY: Ulcerated lesion in anal canal, normal rectal mucosa.

TREATMENT: Following biopsy, lesion was treated with combined chemotherapy and radiation.

PATHOLOGY: Anal squamous cell carcinoma.

ENDORECTAL SONOGRAPHY

Figure 3.7 shows a right posterolateral tumor located in the anal canal occupying nearly half of the circumference. At this level the five sonographic layers of the rectal wall become difficult to visualize and the sphincter muscles become visible instead. The lesion is about 3.5 cm in diameter and appears as a hypoechoic mass with a maximum depth of invasion of nearly 1.5 cm. The tumor appears as a markedly thickened area invading the internal sphincter and there is also possible superficial invasion of the hyperechoic layer corresponding to the external sphincter. There is no evidence of lymph node enlargement.

ANAL SQUAMOUS CELL CARCINOMA

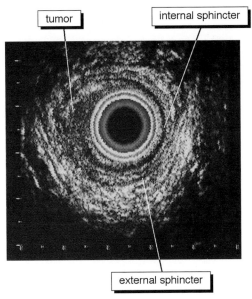

Pre Chemoradiation

Fig. 3.8

TUMOR REGRESSION

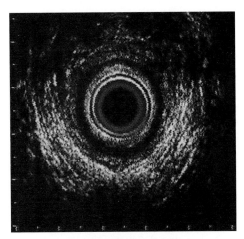

Post Chemoradiation

Fig. 3.9

CLINICAL PRESENTATION

51-yr-old woman presenting with a prolapsing anal lesion associated with bowel movements. These symptoms have been present for 6 months.

PHYSICAL EXAM

INSPECTION: No external lesions seen.
DIGITAL EXAM: Soft polypoid anal lesion palpable on the right side of the anal canal.
SIGMOIDOSCOPY: A 1.5-cm polypoid lesion in the right lateral wall located 1 cm from the anal verge.
TREATMENT: Following biopsy, lesion was treated with combined chemotherapy and radiation.
PATHOLOGY: Anal squamous cell carcinoma.

ENDORECTAL SONOGRAPHY

Figure 3.8 shows a right lateral tumor located in the anal canal occupying nearly 40% of the circumference. The lesion is about 1.5 cm in diameter and appears as a mass with mixed echogenicity extending to a maximum depth of invasion of 0.8 cm. The distal portion of the tumor is seen as a markedly thickened area invading the internal and external sphincters. The more proximal portion of the lesion is located above the level of the sphincters. There are no visible lymph nodes. Figure 3.9 shows complete regression of the tumor following chemoradiation.

Chapter 4

Postsurgical Evaluation

Postsurgical Evaluation

Endorectal sonography is being used frequently as a diagnostic modality in order to obtain follow-up information in patients who had previous endoscopic excision of rectal lesions, as well as in patients who had surgical local excision or wide resection of a rectal tumor with anastomosis. Previous surgical manipulation produces scarring at the site of excision and at the anastomosis which is visible on endorectal sonography and must often be distinguished from recurrent or residual tumor. Following is a series of patients who underwent endorectal sonography at various times after excision of a rectal cancer in order to determine the possible presence of residual or recurrent cancer.

RECTAL WALL

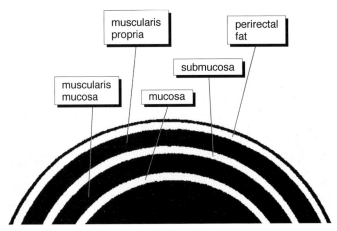

Fig. 4.1

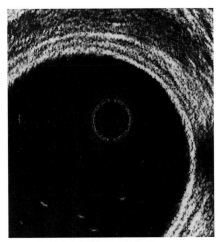

Anatomic Considerations
Fig. 4.2

In order to be able to evaluate rectal lesions, it is necessary to understand the normal sonographic anatomy of the rectal wall. Figure 4.2 compares the five layers of the rectal wall seen on sonography to a schematic drawing (Fig. 4.1). The first hyperechoic layer corresponds to the mucosal interface, the next hypoechoic layer corresponds to the muscularis mucosa, and the middle hyperechoic layer is the submucosal interface. The outer hypoechoic layer is the muscularis propria, and the external hyperechoic layer corresponds to the perirectal fat. Rectal cancer is hypoechoic. Tumor invasion causes destruction of the hyperechoic layers and thickening of the hypoechoic layers.

EVALUATION AFTER EXCISION OF POLYPOID TUMOR

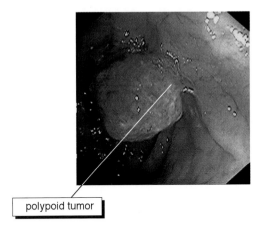

polypoid tumor

Fig. 4.3

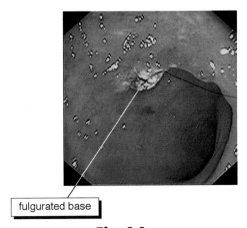

fulgurated base

Fig. 4.4

submucosa

site of excision

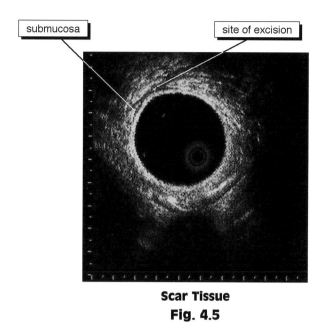

Scar Tissue
Fig. 4.5

CLINICAL PRESENTATION

65-yr-old woman presenting with rectal bleeding. A polypoid rectal lesion was found 8 cm from the anal verge which was excised with a colonoscope 3 months prior to this consultation (Figs. 4.3 and 4.4).

PHYSICAL EXAM

INSPECTION: No external lesions seen.
DIGITAL EXAM: No palpable lesions.
SIGMOIDOSCOPY: No residual lesions seen to 15 cm. Site of excision healed.
PATHOLOGY: Infiltrating, moderately differentiated adenocarcinoma extending to the line of transection.
TREATMENT: Patient advised to be followed with frequent rectal endoscopy and endorectal sonography. Surgery was not recommended because the site of excision was not visible after 3 months and surgery would require a low anterior resection with a possible coloanal anastomosis.
FOLLOW-UP: No evidence of recurrence after 24 months.

ENDORECTAL SONOGRAPHY

Area of thickening approximately 1 cm in diameter and distortion of the layers in the right anterolateral aspect of the rectal wall located 8 cm from the anal verge (Fig. 4.5). The hypoechoic layer corresponding to the muscularis mucosa shows focal widening and there is obliteration of the hyperechoic line corresponding to the submucosa. No lymph nodes are seen. These changes are consistent with postfulguration scar tissue.

EVALUATION AFTER EXCISION OF VILLOUS TUMOR

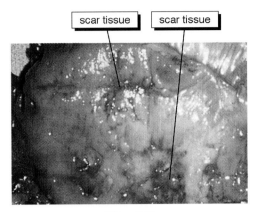

Fig. 4.6

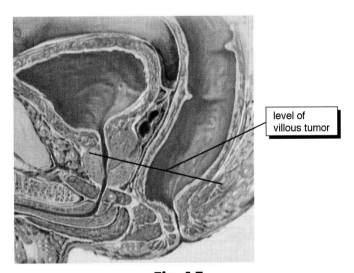

Fig. 4.7

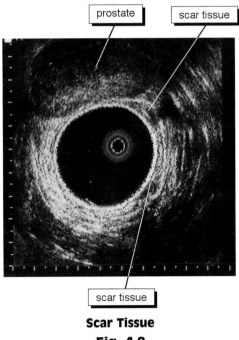

Scar Tissue
Fig. 4.8

CLINICAL PRESENTATION

59-yr-old man who underwent a heart transplant 4 yr ago was found to have a large rectal villous adenoma (8 × 5 cm) with carcinoma in situ. He was treated with a posterior proctotomy 3 months ago. He is now being evaluated for recurrence with one biopsy showing villous adenoma with high-grade dysplasia.

PHYSICAL EXAM

INSPECTION: Mucosal prolapse.
DIGITAL EXAM: Decreased sphincter tone, indurated area present on left side.
SIGMOIDOSCOPY: Raised plaque 2 × 3 cm in size anteriorly on left side at 6 cm from anal verge. Small polypoid lesion 0.5 cm in diameter at 9–10 cm from anal verge (Figs. 4.6 and 4.7).
TREATMENT: In view of the recent biopsy and the sonographic findings, the patient underwent proctectomy with mucosectomy, hand-sewn coloanal anastomosis, and loop ileostomy.
PATHOLOGY: Rectum showing postinflammatory changes, sinus tracts, and foreign body granulomas, no residual tumor.
FOLLOW-UP: No recurrence $2\frac{1}{2}$ yr later.

ENDORECTAL SONOGRAPHY

Two small lesions are seen on the left side, one approximately 1.5 cm in diameter located anteriorly adjacent to the prostate and the other about 1 cm in size located posteriorly at 9 cm from the anal verge (Fig. 4.8). Both lesions are hypoechoic, and there is disruption of the hyperechoic layer which corresponds to the submucosa. The hypoechoic layer representing the muscularis propria is thickened in these two areas and the hyperechoic layer corresponding to the perirectal fat is intact. These two areas may represent postsurgical changes but the presence of recurrent villous tumor and possibly invasive cancer cannot be ruled out.

EVALUATION AFTER EXCISION OF POLYPOID TUMOR

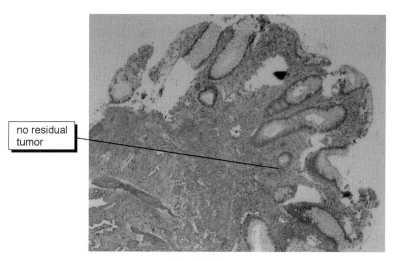

no residual
tumor

Fig. 4.9

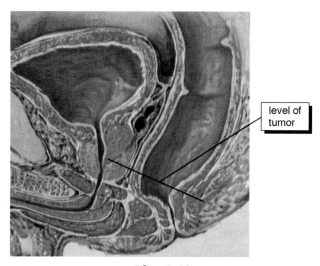

level of
tumor

Fig. 4.10

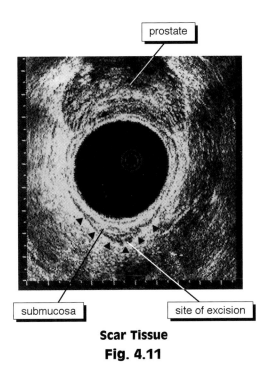

Scar Tissue
Fig. 4.11

CLINICAL PRESENTATION

68-yr-old man who underwent local excision of a 2.5-cm polypoid posterior lesion located at the anorectal junction 12 days ago. The polyp was found to be an adenocarcinoma infiltrating into the submucosa. The margins of excision were close to the tumor.

PHYSICAL EXAM

INSPECTION: Normal.
DIGITAL EXAM: Sutures palpable posteriorly at site of excision of the tumor.
SIGMOIDOSCOPY: Site of tumor resection seen posteriorly at dentate line with residual sutures (Fig. 4.10).
TREATMENT: Transanal re-excision of the previous surgical site with wider lateral and deep margins.
PATHOLOGY: Fragments of anorectal tissue showing acute and chronic inflammation. Skeletal and smooth muscle with fibrosis. No tumor seen (Fig. 4.9).
FOLLOW-UP: No recurrence after 5 yr.

ENDORECTAL SONOGRAPHY

Area of thickening and distortion of the posterior rectal wall and perirectal fat at the level of the prostate, corresponding to the site of previous surgical excision of the tumor (Fig. 4.11). This area occupies nearly 3 cm posteriorly and shows disruption of the hyperechoic submucosal layer with thickening of the hypoechoic layer corresponding to the muscularis propria. The perirectal fat interface appears to be intact (black triangles). There are no visible lymph nodes. These findings are consistent with postsurgical changes caused by edema and fibrosis.

EVALUATION OF STAPLED ANASTOMOSIS

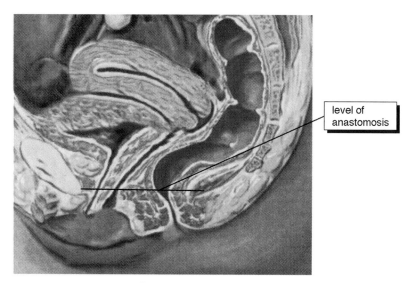

level of anastomosis

Fig. 4.12

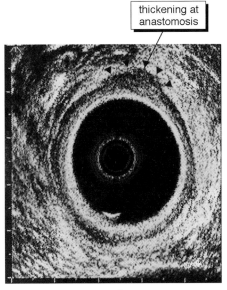

thickening at
anastomosis

Scar Tissue
Fig. 4.13

CLINICAL PRESENTATION

41-yr-old woman who underwent a low anterior resection with everted stapled coloanal anastomosis for a C2 rectal cancer located 6 cm from the anal verge. Patient was subsequently treated with chemoradiotherapy and now returns 6 months after surgery for evaluation.

PHYSICAL EXAM

INSPECTION: Normal.
DIGITAL EXAM: Anastomosis palpable at tip of finger and appears well healed (Fig. 4.12).
SIGMOIDOSCOPY: Anastomosis well healed, rigid pediatric sigmoidoscope passed without difficulty.
FOLLOW-UP: Patient alive and well 5 yr after surgery without evidence of recurrence.

ENDORECTAL SONOGRAPHY

Study performed 6 months after stapled coloanal anastomosis (Fig. 4.13). The sonographic layers of the bowel wall are difficult to distinguish due to scarring from previous surgery and subsequent radiotherapy. There is a localized area of thickening in the left anterolateral portion of the bowel wall at the level of the anastomosis. This area is slightly over 1 cm in diameter and is located in the hypoechoic layer corresponding to the muscularis propria. The area of thickening is also hypoechoic and appears to be originating from the muscularis propria. Although the presence of tumor cannot be ruled out, it appears to represent irregularity of the bowel wall caused by the stapled anastomosis. Follow-up sonograms showed no change, and patient is doing well nearly 5 yr after this study.

INCOMPLETE LOCAL EXCISION FOR CANCER

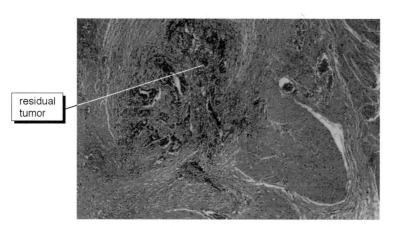

residual
tumor

Fig. 4.14

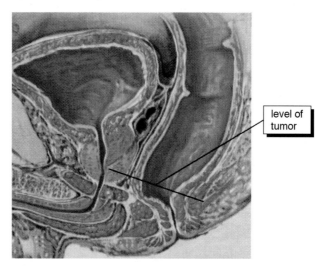

level of
tumor

Fig. 4.15

tumor   prostate

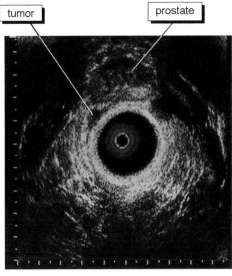

Residual Tumor
Fig. 4.16

CLINICAL PRESENTATION

26-yr-old man with a strong family history of early colorectal cancer who underwent local excision of a polypoid lesion that presented with spontaneous prolapse. The lesion was excised transanally under general anesthesia 3 wk ago and was found to be an infiltrating adenocarcinoma.

PHYSICAL EXAM

INSPECTION: Normal.
DIGITAL EXAM: Hard irregular nodule palpable in right anterolateral rectal wall.
SIGMOIDOSCOPY: Irregular scar tissue present posteriorly at site of previous excision of the tumor at the level of the dentate line. A 1-cm nodule is present at the distal portion of the scar (Fig. 4.15).
TREATMENT: Re-excision of nodule and scar tissue with wider and deeper margins.
PATHOLOGY: Small focus of infiltrating, moderately differentiated adenocarcinoma in smooth muscle wall. Perirectal soft tissue with fibrosis. Margins of resection free of tumor (Fig. 4.14).
FOLLOW-UP: No evidence of recurrence after 30 months.

ENDORECTAL SONOGRAPHY

A 1-cm nodule is present on the right anterior rectal wall at the level of the distal prostate (Fig. 4.16). This lesion is seen to infiltrate the hypoechoic layer corresponding to the internal sphincter, and the more echogenic layer of the external sphincter. At its maximum depth this lesion extends for a distance of 0.8 cm into the rectal wall. There are no visible lymph nodes. These findings are consistent with incomplete previous excision leaving a significant amount of residual tumor.

RECURRENT CANCER AFTER LOCAL EXCISION

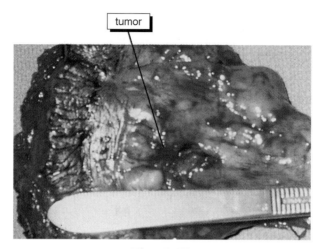

Fig. 4.17

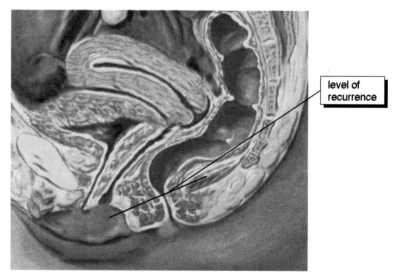

Fig. 4.18

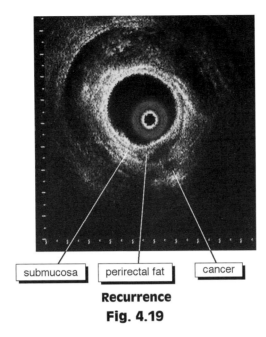

submucosa   perirectal fat   cancer

Recurrence
Fig. 4.19

CLINICAL PRESENTATION

48-yr-old woman who 3 yr ago underwent transanal excision of a villous tumor containing areas of minimally invasive carcinoma. A recurrent benign villous adenoma was excised transanally 1 yr later. The patient now presents with an asymptomatic submucosal 1.5-cm mass at the site of the previous resections.

PHYSICAL EXAM

INSPECTION: Normal.

DIGITAL EXAM: 1.5-cm hard mass palpable in left posterolateral area at the level of the distal rectum and tender to palpation (Fig. 4.18).

SIGMOIDOSCOPY: Submucosal 1.5-cm mass at dentate line without any evidence of ulceration. The mass is located under the scar of previous surgical excision of villous tumor (Fig. 4.17).

TREATMENT: Abdominoperineal resection.

PATHOLOGY: Moderately differentiated adenocarcinoma extending through the rectal adventitia into skeletal muscle. No nodal metastasis seen.

FOLLOW-UP: Patient free of recurrent disease at 3 yr.

ENDORECTAL SONOGRAPHY

Posterior rectal lesion present 0.8 cm in maximal thickness located at dentate line (Fig.4.19). The lesion is hypoechoic and about 1.5 cm in greatest diameter. The hyperechoic submucosal layer is disrupted, the hypoechoic layer corresponding to the muscularis propria is thickened. The tumor extends through the hyperechoic line corresponding to the perirectal fat interface. There are no visible lymph nodes. These findings correspond to those of a deeply infiltrating rectal cancer with invasion to the perirectal fat (uT3, N0).

RECURRENT CANCER AT ANASTOMOSIS

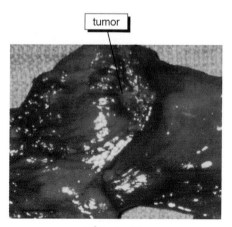

Fig. 4.20

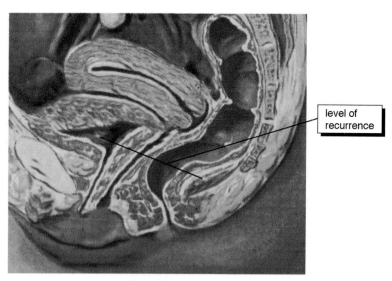

Fig. 4.21

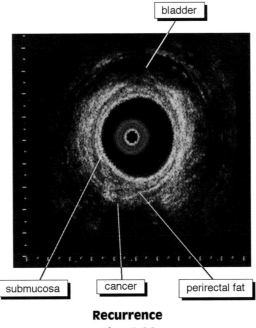

Recurrence
Fig. 4.22

CLINICAL PRESENTATION

56-yr-old woman who underwent an anterior resection for a Dukes' B1 rectal cancer located 11 cm from the anal verge 21 months ago. She was found to have an asymptomatic recurrence at the anastomosis on routine follow-up.

PHYSICAL EXAM

INSPECTION: Normal.
DIGITAL EXAM: No palpable lesion.
SIGMOIDOSCOPY: Ulcerated lesion located posteriorly 9 cm from the anal verge at the site of the previous anastomosis (Figs. 4.20 and 4.21).
TREATMENT: Low anterior resection with mucosectomy and hand-sewn coloanal anastomosis.
PATHOLOGY: Moderately differentiated adenocarcinoma at anastomotic line with transmural invasion into perirectal soft tissue. No nodal metastasis seen.
FOLLOW-UP: No evidence of recurrence at $2\frac{1}{2}$ yr.

ENDORECTAL SONOGRAPHY

Lesion seen in the right posterolateral aspect of the rectum at 9 cm from the anal verge (Fig. 4.22). It is about 2 cm in diameter and 0.8 cm in depth. The sonographic layers of the bowel wall are difficult to see clearly due to scarring from previous surgery. The hyperechoic submucosal line appears to be disrupted and there is thickening of the hypoechoic layer corresponding to the muscularis propria. The perirectal fat interface is irregular and shows focal areas of disruption consistent with tumor invasion. There are no visible lymph nodes. These findings correspond to those seen with a deeply infiltrating tumor invading into the perirectal fat (uT3, N0).

RECURRENT CANCER AT ANASTOMOSIS

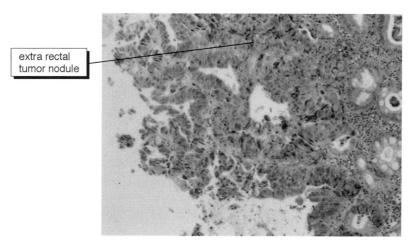

extra rectal
tumor nodule

Fig. 4.23

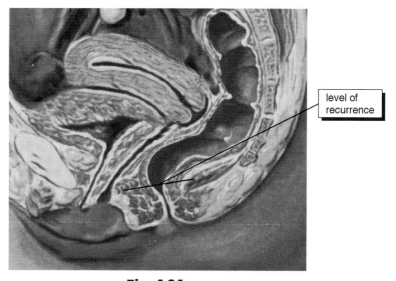

level of
recurrence

Fig. 4.24

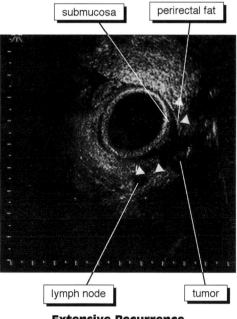

| submucosa | perirectal fat |

| lymph node | tumor |

Extensive Recurrence
Fig. 4.25

CLINICAL PRESENTATION

72-yr-old woman who 30 months ago had a pelvic exenteration for rectal cancer with invasion of the cervix and uterus. She now presents with a recurrence at the colorectal anastomosis which on biopsy is reported as moderately differentiated adenocarcinoma. She received a course of 4,500 cGy to the pelvis prior to this evaluation.

PHYSICAL EXAM

INSPECTION: Normal.
DIGITAL EXAM: Hard, ulcerated lesion at about 6 cm fixed to the sacrum (Fig. 4.24).
SIGMOIDOSCOPY: Lesion as described above, ulcerated, located posteriorly 6 cm from the anal verge at the level of the previous anastomosis. The lesion is fixed to the sacrum.
TREATMENT: Exploratory laparotomy with end sigmoid colostomy.
PATHOLOGY: Unresectable, moderately differentiated adenocarcinoma with invasion of the sacrum and lateral pelvic wall with nodal metastasis (Fig. 4.23).

ENDORECTAL SONOGRAPHY

Left posterolateral ulcerated lesion located 6 cm from the anal verge at the site of the previous colorectal anastomosis (Fig. 4.25). The tumor occupies one-third of the rectal circumference and penetrates deeply beyond the bowel wall. The various layers of the bowel wall are not well seen due to scarring from previous surgery and subsequent radiotherapy. Several hypoechoic enlarged lymph nodes are present adjacent to the tumor. These findings are consistent with an advanced recurrent tumor, invading deeply beyond the bowel wall to the pelvic sidewall, with multiple nodal metastasis.

Chapter 5
Effect of Radiotherapy

Effect of Radiotherapy

Radiotherapy is used frequently in the pre- and postoperative treatment of patients with advanced rectal cancer. Also, occasionally, patients with previous radiotherapy for other pelvic malignancies develop rectal cancer and require endorectal sonographic evaluation. The effect of previous radiation is to blur the echogenic distinctions of the layers of the bowel wall. Evaluation of patients who have received preoperative chemoradiotherapy for advanced rectal cancer often shows significant tumor regression. Accurate staging following radiation is more difficult since scarring and edema may lead to overstaging of the residual tumor.

PREVIOUS RADIOTHERAPY FOR CERVICAL CANCER

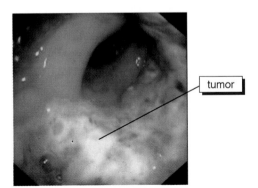

tumor

Fig. 5.1

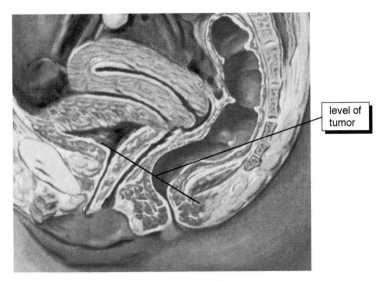

level of
tumor

Fig. 5.2

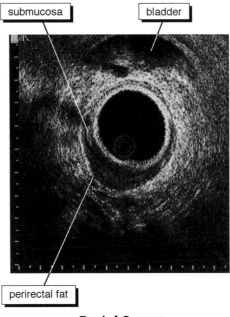

submucosa   bladder

perirectal fat

Rectal Cancer
Fig. 5.3

CLINICAL PRESENTATION

53-yr-old woman who was treated with radiotherapy for cervical cancer 5 yr ago and now was found to have a palpable rectal tumor on follow-up physical exam.

PHYSICAL EXAM

INSPECTION: Skin over the sacrum and lower abdomen shows postradiation changes.
DIGITAL EXAM: Stricture of anorectal sphincter and palpable ulcerated tumor in the right posterolateral rectal wall.
SIGMOIDOSCOPY: Ulcerated 2 × 2 cm tumor with lower margin at the dentate line (Figs. 5.1 and 5.2).
TREATMENT: Abdominoperineal resection.
PATHOLOGY: Moderately differentiated adenocarcinoma with colloid features extending to the junction of the rectal wall and perirectal fat. No nodal metastasis seen. Right lateral margin of resection showed dense fibrosis with a fragment of carcinoma which is not seen on sonography.
FOLLOW-UP: Biopsy of abdominal wall nodule 3 yr later showed metastatic adenocarcinoma.

ENDORECTAL SONOGRAPHY

A 4-cm lesion located 6 cm from the anal verge is present (Fig. 5.3). The tumor is 1.5 cm in thickness. The layers of the bowel wall are somewhat difficult to distinguish due to the previous radiotherapy. The hyperechoic layer representing the submucosa is destroyed and there is thickening of the hypoechoic layer corresponding to the muscularis propria consistent with tumor invasion. The hyperechoic line representing the perirectal fat interface appears to be intact. There are no visible lymph nodes. These findings are consistent with a tumor invading deeply into the muscularis propria with negative nodes (uT2,N0).

RESIDUAL RECTAL CANCER AFTER RADIOTHERAPY

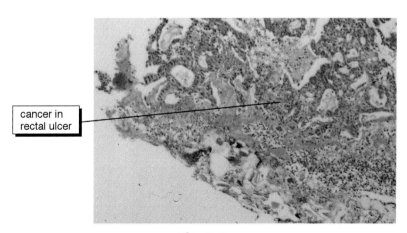

cancer in
rectal ulcer

Fig. 5.4

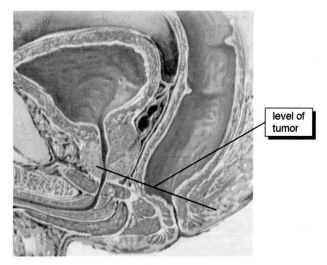

level of
tumor

Fig. 5.5

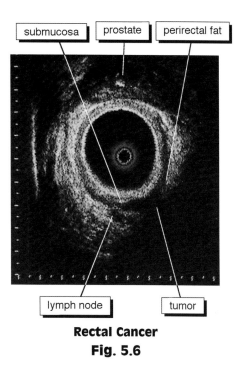

submucosa | prostate | perirectal fat

lymph node | tumor

Rectal Cancer
Fig. 5.6

CLINICAL PRESENTATION

70-yr-old man with a distal rectal cancer previously treated with fulguration followed by chemoradiation.

PHYSICAL EXAM

INSPECTION: Some edema and induration of perianal skin.

DIGITAL EXAM: Area of induration and ulceration in the distal rectum posteriorly.

SIGMOIDOSCOPY: Superficial ulceration starting just above the level of the dentate line posteriorly, surrounded by area of induration (Fig. 5.5).

TREATMENT: Biopsy of ulcerated area.

PATHOLOGY: Moderately differentiated adenocarcinoma (Fig. 5.4).

FOLLOW-UP: Patient refused abdominopherineal resection.

ENDORECTAL SONOGRAPHY

Shows destruction of the hyperechoic line that corresponds to the submucosal layer and thickening of the hypoechoic layer corresponding to the muscularis propria in the distal rectum along the left posterolateral aspect of the rectal circumference (Fig. 5.6). This thickening occupies about half of the rectal circumference and is 0.5 cm at its maximum depth. The layers of the bowel wall are not well seen due to previous radiotherapy. There is loss of the hyperechoic layer that corresponds to the perirectal fat interface at the apex of the lesion consistent with tumor invasion. An enlarged lymph node is seen posteriorly which is 0.7 cm in diameter and hypoechoic. This appearance and size correlates with a high probability of lymph node metastasis. These findings indicate residual tumor with deep invasion into the perirectal fat and nodal metastasis.

RESIDUAL CANCER AFTER RADIOTHERAPY

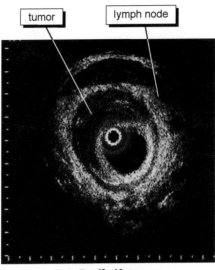

Pre Radiotherapy

Fig. 5.7

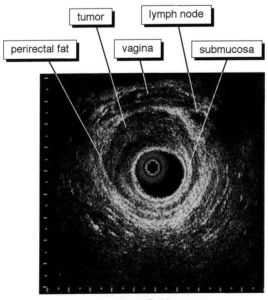

Post Radiotherapy

Fig. 5.8

CLINICAL PRESENTATION

31-yr-old woman who presents with an advanced rectal cancer. The patient underwent chemoradiation prior to surgical treatment.

PHYSICAL EXAM

INSPECTION: Minimal perianal edema.

DIGITAL EXAM: Extensive tumor located mostly on the right side with significant narrowing of the lumen.

SIGMOIDOSCOPY: Large friable cancer starting at level of dentate line.

TREATMENT: Abdominoperineal resection with excision of posterior vaginal wall.

PATHOLOGY: Colloid carcinoma infiltrating the perirectal fat and lymphatics. There is tumor in the rectovaginal septum. Five lymph nodes have metastatic disease. The tumor extends to the right lateral surgical margin.

FOLLOW-UP: This patient expired 18 months after surgery.

ENDORECTAL SONOGRAPHY

Sonogram obtained prior to preoperative chemoradiation shows a large rectal tumor located in the right anterolateral wall and occupying more than half of the rectal circumference (Fig. 5.7). The lesion has a maximum thickness of 2 cm. There is obliteration of the hyperechoic layer corresponding to the submucosa and marked thickening of the hypoechoic layer representing the muscularis propria consistent with tumor invasion. The hyperechoic layer corresponding to the perirectal fat interface also appears invaded by tumor. The tumor is very close to the posterior vaginal wall and there may be invasion into the rectovaginal septum. Multiple large (0.5–1.0 cm) hypoechoic lymph nodes are present consistent with tumor invasion. There is no regression of the tumor following chemoradiation and the lymph node that is labeled appears to have increased in size (Fig. 5.8).

TUMOR REGRESSION AFTER RADIATION

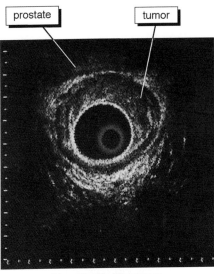

Pre Radiotherapy

Fig. 5.9

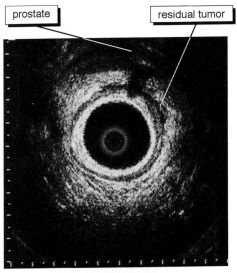

Post Radiotherapy

Fig. 5.10

CLINICAL PRESENTATION

53-yr-old man who presents with an advanced rectal cancer. Symptoms include rectal bleeding, tenesmus, and pencil thin stools. The patient underwent chemoradiation prior to surgical treatment with marked tumor regression.

PHYSICAL EXAM

INSPECTION: Small external hemorrhoids.

DIGITIAL EXAM: Large, hard, fixed circumferential lesion located just above the dentate line.

SIGMOIDOSCOPY: Circumferential cancer 6 cm from the anal verge with significant narrowing of the lumen.

TREATMENT: Low anterior resection with mucosectomy and hand-sewn J-pouch-anal anastomosis.

PATHOLOGY: Moderately differentiated residual adenocarcinoma invading the submusosa. Lymph nodes are negative.

FOLLOW-UP: This patient developed lung metastasis 1 year later.

ENDORECTAL SONOGRAPHY

Sonogram before chemoradiation shows a large circumferential rectal tumor (Fig. 5.9). The lesion has a maximum thickness of 1.5 cm. There is loss of the hyperechoic layer corresponding to the submucosa and marked thickening of the hypoechoic layer corresponding to the muscularis propria consistent with tumor invasion. The hyperechoic layer representing the perirectal fat interface is irregular and in one image the tumor appears to invade the prostatic capsule. Three hypoechoic lymph nodes 0.4 to 0.5 cm in diameter are present proximal to the tumor (not shown). Three months later, following chemoradiation, there is only a 2-cm area of residual tumor in the left anterolateral rectal wall. The previously seen lymph nodes are no longer present (Fig. 5.10).

Chapter 6
Villous Adenoma

Villous Adenoma

Sonographic evaluation of a villous rectal lesion is helpful in determining the presence of tumor invasion. Villous lesions are often bulky and difficult to evaluate. The presence of an intact hyperechoic submucosal interface indicates lack of tumor invasion into the submucosa. In large carpeting lesions, careful evaluation of the entire tumor is necessary to determine that a small area of invasion has not been overlooked. In benign villous lesions, there should not be any enlarged perirectal nodes. Presence of lymphadenopathy should alert the examiner that malignant degeneration with lymphatic metastasis is possible and excision of the rectal segment with perirectal nodes may be indicated as opposed to local excision.

VILLOUS ADENOMA

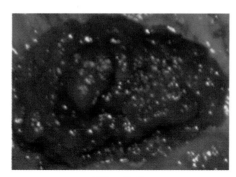

Fig. 6.1

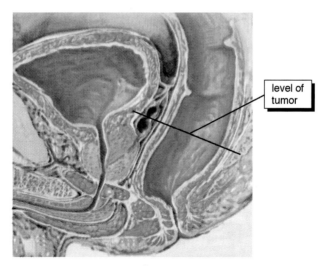

Fig. 6.2

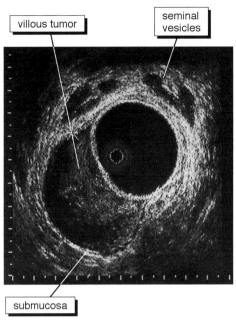

Benign Villous Adenoma
Fig. 6.3

CLINICAL PRESENTATION

58-yr-old man presenting with a 2-yr history of rectal bleeding.

PHYSICAL EXAM

INSPECTION: Prolapsed hemorrhoids.

DIGITAL EXAM: No palpable masses.

SIGMOIDOSCOPY: Large polypoid lesion seen 11 cm from the anal verge (Figs. 6.1 and 6.2).

TREATMENT: Low anterior resection with stapled colorectal anastomosis.

PATHOLOGY: Large polypoid tumor 6 by 3 cm in diameter. The tumor is a tubulovillous adenoma with a segment of well-differentiated adenocarcinoma invading the submucosa. There is no tumor in the lymph nodes.

FOLLOW-UP: No recurrence at 3 yr.

ENDORECTAL SONOGRAPHY

Large polypoid rectal tumor occupying 40% of the rectal circumference in the right posterolateral aspect and located at the level of the seminal vesicles (Fig. 6.3). The tumor is 6 cm in greatest diameter and about 3 cm in thickness. The hyperechoic submucosal interface is intact surrounding the lesion consistent with a benign villous adenoma. In one sonographic view, not shown, the submucosal line is interrupted consistent with tumor invasion of the submucosa. There are no visible lymph nodes. These findings correspond to those of a villous adenoma with a small area of cancer invading the submucosa.

VILLOUS ADENOMA?

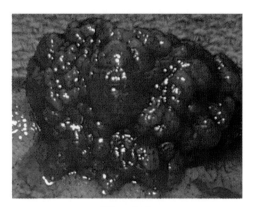

Fig. 6.4

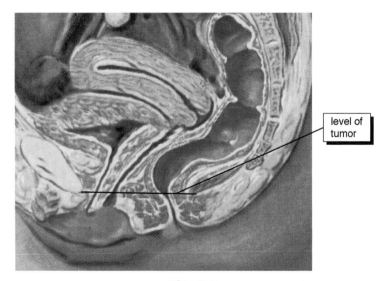

Fig. 6.5

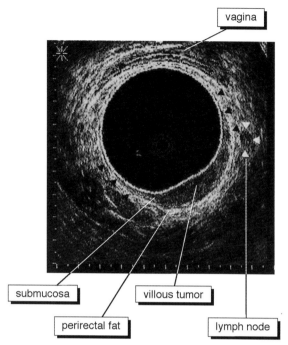

Dukes' A Carcinoma
Fig. 6.6

CLINICAL PRESENTATION

57-yr-old woman with 1-yr history of passage of mucus and blood with bowel movements.

PHYSICAL EXAM

INSPECTION: No external lesions seen.

DIGITAL EXAM: Soft villous tumor palpable posteriorly at the dentate line without evidence of induration (Fig. 6.4).

SIGMOIDOSCOPY: Villous tumor present 4 to 9 cm from the anal verge in the posterior rectal wall (Fig. 6.5).

TREATMENT: Full-thickness excision via posterior proctotomy.

PATHOLOGY: Sessile tubulovillous adenoma containing moderately differentiated adenocarcinoma with colloid features. The tumor infiltrates the submucosa. Lymph nodes are free of tumor.

FOLLOW-UP: The tumor recurred 3 yr later and the patient underwent a proctectomy with hand-sewn coloanal anastomosis.

ENDORECTAL SONOGRAPHY

Tumor present in the posterior rectal wall starting just above the dentate line and extending to 9 cm from the anal verge (Fig. 6.6). The lesion occupies 40% of the rectal circumference and has the appearance of a benign villous adenoma in most of the sections. In the section shown, the hyperechoic line corresponding to the submucosal layer is interrupted consistent with tumor invasion. There is no thickening of the hypoechoic layer corresponding to the muscularis propria, and the hyperechoic layer corresponding to the perirectal fat interface is intact. A small lymph node 0.5 cm in diameter is present with the appearance of a benign hyperplatic node. These findings represent a Dukes A lesion arising in a villous adenoma.

Chapter 7

Submucosal Invasion

Submucosal Invasion

Submucosal invasion is diagnosed by disruption of the hyperechoic submucosal interface. The tumor is hypoechoic, and invasion of the submucosa results in destruction of the hyperechoic line that represents the submucosal layer. This layer is usually well seen and its disruption is a reliable sign of tumor invasion. Accurate preoperative staging of early cancers is important if local excision is to be considered a treatment alternative. Evaluation of associated perirectal nodes is also important since up to 14% of tumors with submucosal invasion may have nodal metastasis and therefore require proctectomy instead of local excision.

pT1

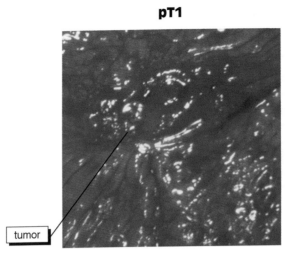

Fig. 7.1

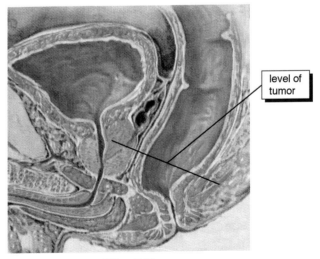

Fig. 7.2

uT1

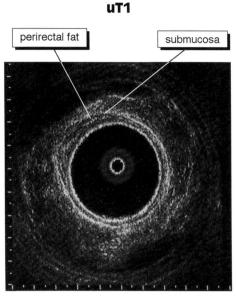

perirectal fat

submucosa

Fig. 7.3

CLINICAL PRESENTATION

68-yr-old man found to have a small asymptomatic tumor in the rectum while undergoing sigmoidoscopy during a routine physical exam.

PHYSICAL EXAM

INSPECTION: No abnormalities seen.

DIGITAL EXAM: No palpable lesions.

SIGMOIDOSCOPY: Small flat tumor present 8 cm from the anal verge, located on the right anterior rectal wall (Fig. 7.1 and 7.2).

TREATMENT: Low anterior resection with mucosectomy and hand-sewn coloanal anastomosis.

PATHOLOGY: Moderately differentiated adenocarcinoma invading the submucosa. There is no tumor in the lymph nodes.

FOLLOW-UP: No recurrence at $2\frac{1}{2}$ yr.

ENDORECTAL SONOGRAPHY

Tumor located in the right anterior rectal wall 8 cm from the anal verge (Fig. 7.3). The lesion is approximately 3 cm in diameter and 0.7 cm in depth. The hyperechoic layer corresponding to the submucosa is interrupted at several points consistent with tumor invasion. The hypoechoic layer representing the muscularis propria is intact as is the hyperechoic layer corresponding to the perirectal fat interface. There are no visible perirectal lymph nodes. These findings correspond to a Dukes A tumor.

pT1

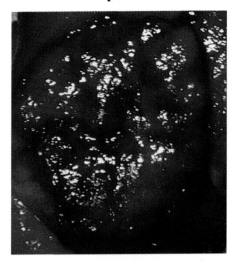

Fig. 7.4

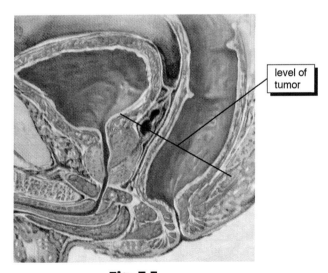

level of
tumor

Fig. 7.5

uT1

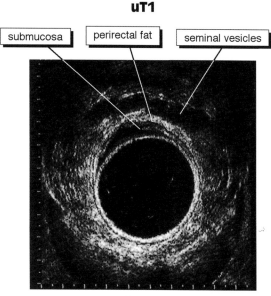

submucosa | perirectal fat | seminal vesicles

Fig. 7.6

CLINICAL PRESENTATION

55-yr-old man who presented with rectal bleeding.

PHYSICAL EXAM

INSPECTION: No abnormalities seen.

DIGITAL EXAM: Movable hard lesion with overhanging edges palpable at fingertip.

SIGMOIDOSCOPY: Friable tumor present 7 cm from the anal verge, about 3 cm in diameter with central ulceration. Lesion is located in right anterolateral rectal wall (Fig. 7.4 and 7.5).

TREATMENT: Low anterior resection with everted double-stapled coloanal anastomosis.

PATHOLOGY: Moderately differentiated adenocarcinoma invading the submuscosa. Lymph nodes are free of tumor.

FOLLOW-UP: Patient is doing well 4 yr after surgery.

ENDORECTAL SONOGRAPHY

Shows a 3-cm tumor located in the right anterolateral rectal wall (Fig. 7.6). The lesion is 0.8 cm in depth and is located at the level of the seminal vesicles. The hyperechoic layer corresponding to the submucosa is interrupted consistent with tumor invasion. There is only minimal thickening of the hypoechoic layer corresponding to the muscularis propria, and the hyperechoic layer that represents the perirectal fat interface is intact. There are no visible lymph nodes. These findings correspond to those of a Dukes A lesion.

pT1

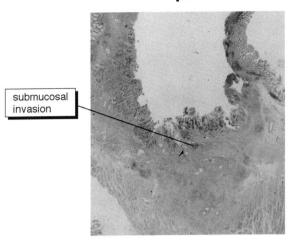

submucosal invasion

Fig. 7.7

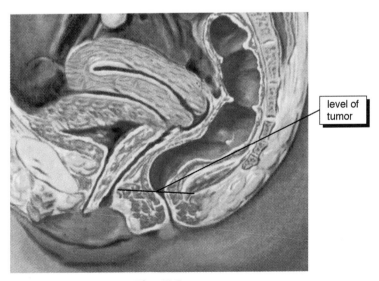

level of tumor

Fig. 7.8

uT1

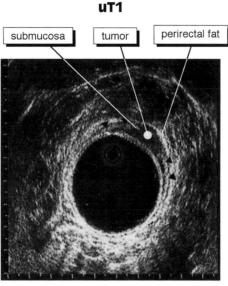

submucosa | tumor | perirectal fat

Fig. 7.9

CLINICAL PRESENTATION

42-yr-old woman presenting with a 1-yr history of rectal bleeding originally attributed to hemorrhoids.

PHYSICAL EXAM

INSPECTION: No abnormalities seen.

DIGITAL EXAM: Hard mass with central ulceration palpable anteriorly.

SIGMOIDOSCOPY: 3-cm ulcerated tumor located 5 cm from the anal verge is present in the anterior rectal wall.

TREATMENT: Abdominoperineal resection.

PATHOLOGY: Moderately differentiated rectal adenocarcinoma infiltrating the submucosa (Fig. 7.7). There is no tumor in the lymph nodes.

FOLLOW-UP: Patient is well 5 yr after surgery.

ENDORECTAL SONOGRAPHY

Shows a 3-cm lesion located anteriorly 5 cm from the anal verge (Fig. 7.8). The tumor is 0.9 cm in depth. The hyperechoic layer corresponding to the submucosa is interrupted consistent with tumor invasion (Fig. 7.9); the hypoechoic layer representing the muscularis propria and the hyperechoic layer that represents the perirectal fat interface are intact. There are no visible lymph nodes. These findings correspond to those seen in a Dukes A tumor.

Chapter 8

Invasion of Muscular Layer

Invasion of Muscular Layer

Sonographic diagnosis of tumor invasion of the muscularis propria is based on thickening of this layer. The muscularis propria is represented by a thin hypoechoic layer adjacent to the hyperechoic submucosal interface. Since the tumor is also hypoechoic, early muscular invasion is difficult to detect. In Dukes' B1 lesions, the submucosal interface is disrupted and the muscularis propria is significantly thicker than the adjacent normal layers. The surrounding hyperechoic layer corresponding to the perirectal fat interface remains intact and there should be no lymphadenopathy.

pT2

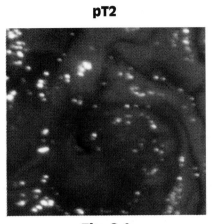

Fig. 8.1

focal muscle invasion

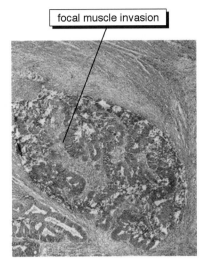

Fig. 8.2

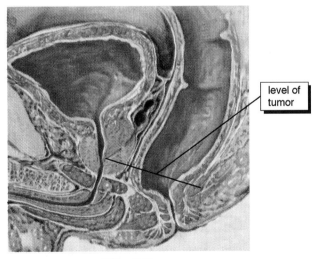

level of
tumor

Fig. 8.3

uT1

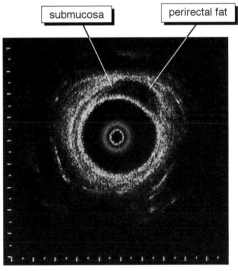

submucosa   perirectal fat

Fig. 8.4

CLINICAL PRESENTATION

60-yr-old man found to have a polypoid rectal cancer on surveillance colonoscopy at the site of previous endoscopic excision of a benign villous lesion.

PHYSICAL EXAM

INSPECTION: No lesions seen.

DIGITAL EXAM: Friable polypoid lesion with central ulceration palpable on the anterior rectal wall.

SIGMOIDOSCOPY: Tumor located 6 cm from the anal verge on the anterior rectal wall (Fig. 8.1).

TREATMENT: Low anterior resection with mucosectomy and hand-sewn coloanal anastomosis.

PATHOLOGY: Moderately differentiated rectal adenocarcinoma invading the muscularis propria (Fig. 8.2). Lymph nodes are negative for tumor.

FOLLOW-UP: Patient is well 3 yr later.

ENDORECTAL SONOGRAPHY

There is a 3-cm tumor occupying the anterior hemicircumference of the rectal wall located 6 cm from the anal verge (Fig. 8.3). The tumor is 1.0 cm in thickness. The hyperechoic layer corresponding to the submucosa is interrupted consistent with tumor invasion (Fig. 8.4). The hypoechoic layer corresponding to the muscularis propria is slightly thickened in only one section. The hyperechoic layer representing the perirectal fat is intact. There are no visible lymph nodes. This study was originally reported as consistent with a Dukes A lesion. Histologic examination of the tumor shows focal invasion of the muscularis propria which is not evident on the sonogram. There are no visible lymph nodes.

pT2

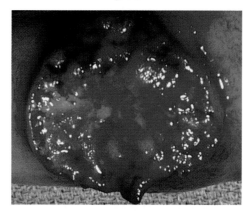

Fig. 8.5

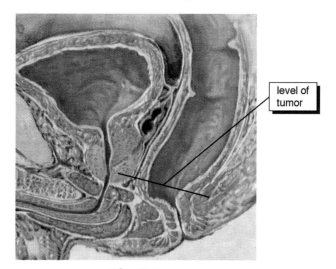

level of
tumor

Fig. 8.6

uT2

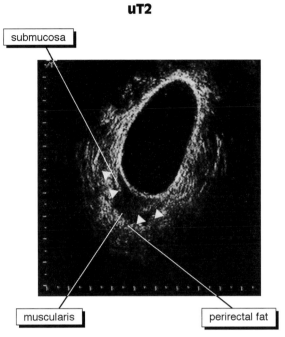

Fig. 8.7

CLINICAL PRESENTATION

61-yr-old man presenting with rectal bleeding initially attributed to hemorrhoids.

PHYSICAL EXAM

INSPECTION: No abnormalities seen.

DIGITAL EXAM: No palpable lesions.

SIGMOIDOSCOPY: Internal hemorrhoids. Ulcerated tumor seen 10 cm from the anal verge occupying one-third of the rectal circumference (Fig. 8.5).

TREATMENT: Low anterior resection with everted double-stapled coloanal anastomosis.

PATHOLOGY: Moderately differentiated adenocarcinoma invading the muscularis propria. Lymph nodes are free of tumor.

FOLLOW-UP: Patient is doing well 4 yr postoperatively.

ENDORECTAL SONOGRAPHY

Shows a 3.5-cm lesion located 10 cm from the anal verge and nearly 1.5 cm in depth (Fig. 8.6). The hyperechoic layer corresponding to the submucosa is interrupted consistent with tumor invasion (Fig. 8.7). The hypoechoic layer that represents the muscularis propria is significantly thickened due to tumor invasion. The hyperechoic layer corresponding to the perirectal fat interface is intact. There are no visible lymph nodes. These findings are consistent with a Dukes B1 lesion.

pT2

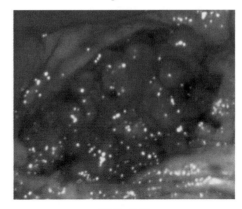

Fig. 8.8

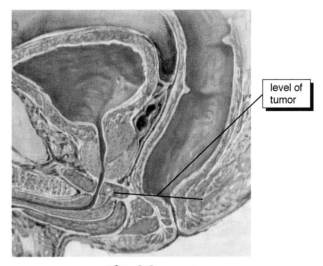

level of
tumor

Fig. 8.9

uT2

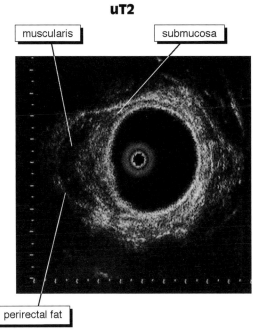

muscularis submucosa

perirectal fat

Fig. 8.10

CLINICAL PRESENTATION

70-yr-old man with long history of rectal bleeding from hemorrhoids found to have a rectal tumor on routine sigmoidoscopy.

PHYSICAL EXAM

INSPECTION: No lesions seen.

DIGITAL EXAM: Polypoid tumor with hard border and central ulceration palpable in the right lateral rectal wall (Fig. 8.8).

SIGMOIDOSCOPY: 3 × 3 cm lesion located 5 cm from the anal verge.

TREATMENT: Abdominoperineal resection.

PATHOLOGY: Moderately differentiated adenocarcinoma invading the muscularis propria. No tumor is seen in the lymph nodes.

FOLLOW-UP: Patient is well 3 yr postoperatively.

ENDORECTAL SONOGRAPHY

Rectal tumor located 5 cm from the anal verge 4.5 cm in diameter and occupying the right lateral rectal wall (Fig. 8.9). The thickness of the tumor is about 2.5 cm. The hyperechoic layer corresponding to the submucosa is infiltrated and the hypoechoic layer corresponding to the muscularis propria is markedly thickened consistent with tumor invasion (Fig. 8.10). The hyperechoic layer representing the perirectal fat interface is intact. There are no visible lymph nodes. These findings correspond to those of a Dukes B1 lesion.

pT2

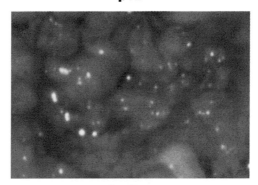

Fig. 8.11

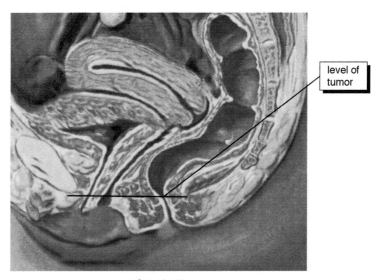

level of
tumor

Fig. 8.12

uT2

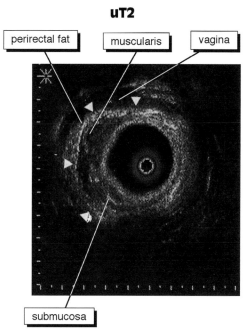

perirectal fat | muscularis | vagina

submucosa

Fig. 8.13

CLINICAL PRESENTATION

54-yr-old woman who presented with rectal bleeding, constipation, and passage of pencil thin stools.

PHYSICAL EXAM

INSPECTION: No abnormalities seen.

DIGITAL EXAM: Hard, movable lesion with central ulceration, located in the distal rectum (Fig. 8.11).

SIGMOIDOSCOPY: Lesion at 5 cm occupying the right lateral rectal wall, arising at the dentate line and extending proximally for a length of 6 cm (Fig. 8.12).

TREATMENT: Abdominoperineal resection with excision of the posterior vaginal wall.

PATHOLOGY: Moderately differentiated adenocarcinoma infiltrating the muscularis propria. Lymph nodes are free of metastasis.

FOLLOW-UP: Patient is doing well 3 yr after surgery.

ENDORECTAL SONOGRAPHY

Tumor 5 cm from the anal verge occupying the entire right hemicircumference with extension anteriorly (Fig. 8.13). The lesion is approximately 4.5 cm in diameter and 1.2 cm in depth. The hyperechoic layer corresponding to the submucosa is destroyed and the hypoechoic layer representing the muscularis propria is thickened consistent with tumor invasion. The hyperechoic layer which corresponds to the perirectal fat interface is intact. The tumor is close to the posterior vaginal wall but there is no sonographic evidence of invasion. There are no visible lymph nodes. These findings correspond to those of a Dukes B1 lesion.

pT2

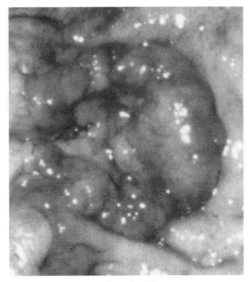

Fig. 8.14

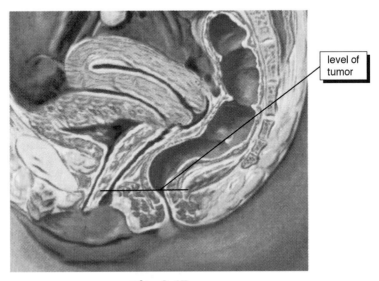

level of tumor

Fig. 8.15

uT2

muscularis | vagina | submucosa

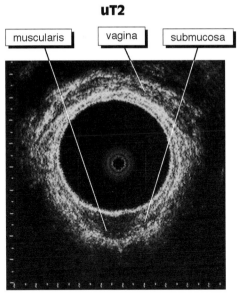

Fig. 8.16

CLINICAL PRESENTATION

66-yr-old woman presenting with a 1-month history of rectal bleeding without change in bowel habits.

PHYSICAL EXAM

INSPECTION: Unremarkable.

DIGITAL EXAM: Hard movable posterior lesion with central ulceration (Fig. 8.14).

SIGMOIDOSCOPY: Posterior lesion located 5 cm from the anal verge, 3 cm in diameter. The lower border of the tumor starts just above the dentate line (Fig. 8.15).

TREATMENT: Abdominoperineal resection.

PATHOLOGY: Moderately differentiated adenocarcinoma infiltrating the muscularis propria. Lymph nodes are negative for tumor.

FOLLOW-UP: Patient is well 3 yrs postoperatively.

ENDORECTAL SONOGRAPHY

Shows a 3-cm tumor in the posterior rectal wall 5 cm from the anal verge (Fig. 8.16). The lesion is 1.5 cm in depth. The hyperechoic layer corresponding to the submucosa is destroyed and the hypoechoic layer corresponding to the muscularis propria is thickened consistent with tumor invasion. The hyperechoic layer which represents the perirectal fat interface is intact. There are no visible lymph nodes. These findings correspond to those of a Dukes B1 lesion.

pT2

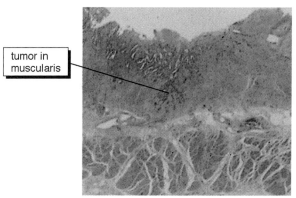

tumor in muscularis

Fig. 8.17

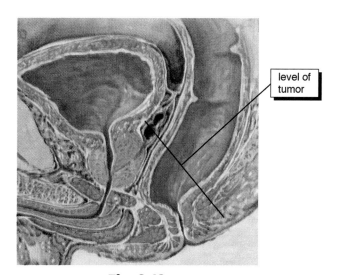

level of tumor

Fig. 8.18

uT2

muscularis   seminal
                  vesicles   submucosa

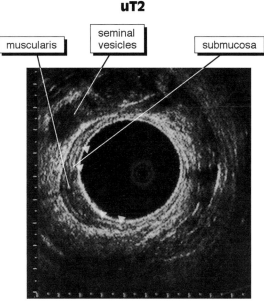

Fig. 8.19

CLINICAL PRESENTATION

78-yr-old man presenting with rectal bleeding for 8 months.

PHYSICAL EXAM

INSPECTION: Unremarkable.

DIGITAL EXAM: Ulcerated hard lesion occupying about half the rectal circumference palpable posteriorly.

SIGMOIDOSCOPY: Ulcerated tumor located 6 cm from the anal verge in the right posterolateral aspect of the rectum (Fig. 8.18).

TREATMENT: Abdominoperineal resection.

PATHOLOGY: Moderately differentiated adenocarcinoma with superficial muscular invasion. Lymph nodes are free of tumor (Fig. 8.17).

FOLLOW-UP: This patient is asymptomatic 4 yr after surgery.

ENDORECTAL SONOGRAPHY

There is a 5-cm tumor 6 cm from the anal verge at the level of the prostate and seminal vesicles (Fig. 8.19). The lesion is located in the right posterolateral wall and encompasses half of the rectal circumference. The tumor is 1 cm at its maximal thickness. The hyperechoic layer corresponding to the submucosa is destroyed and the hypoechoic layer representing the muscularis propria is thickened consistent with tumor invasion. The outer hyperechoic layer which corresponds to the perirectal fat interface is intact. There are no visible lymph nodes. These findings correspond to those of a Dukes B1 tumor.

pT2

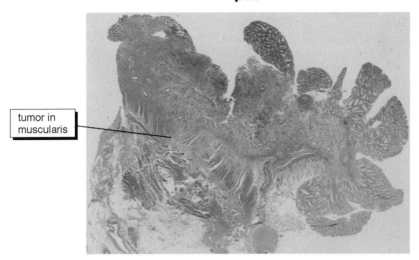

Fig. 8.20

tumor in
muscularis

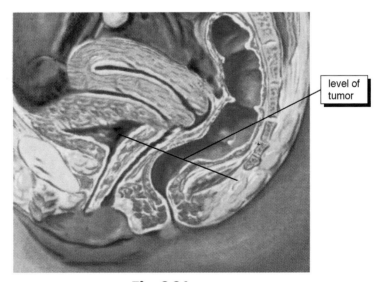

level of
tumor

Fig. 8.21

uT2

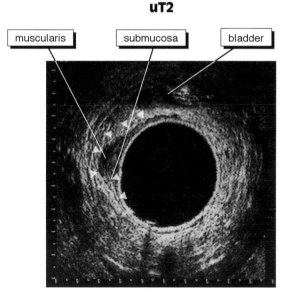

Fig. 8.22

CLINICAL PRESENTATION

55-yr-old woman being evaluated for rectal bleeding.

PHYSICAL EXAM

INSPECTION: Unremarkable.

DIGITAL EXAM: No tumor palpable.

SIGMOIDOSCOPY: Small ulcerated polypoid tumor located 10–11 cm from the anal verge (Fig. 8.21).

TREATMENT: Anterior resection with stapled anastomosis.

PATHOLOGY: Moderately differentiated adenocarcinoma associated with a tubulovillous adenoma. The tumor invades the muscularis propria (Fig. 8.20). Lymph nodes are free of tumor.

FOLLOW-UP: This patient had a recurrence at the colorectal anastomosis 21 months later. She underwent a secondary low anterior resection with mucosectomy and hand-sewn coloanal anastomosis. She is doing well 2 yrs postoperatively.

ENDORECTAL SONOGRAPHY

Sonography shows a 2.5-cm tumor located in the right lateral rectal wall 10 cm from the anal verge (Fig. 8.22). The lesion is 1.5 cm in greatest depth and the anterior border appears to be a villous adenoma. The central portion shows destruction of the hyperechoic layer representing the submucosa and thickening of the hypoechoic layer corresponding to the muscularis. These findings represent tumor invasion. In the villous portion of the tumor these layers remain intact. The hyperechoic layer corresponding to the perirectal far interface is intact. There are no visible lymph nodes. These findings correspond to those of a Dukes B1 cancer arising in a villous adenoma.

pT2

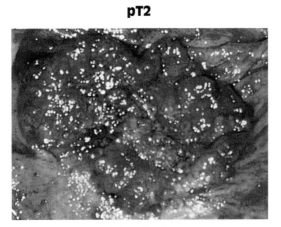

Fig. 8.23

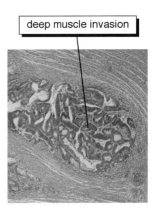

deep muscle invasion

Fig. 8.24

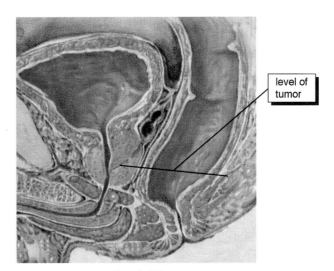

level of tumor

Fig. 8.25

uT3

invasion ?   muscularis   perirectal fat

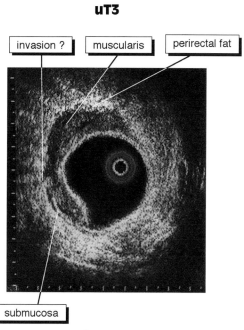

submucosa

Fig. 8.26

CLINICAL PRESENTATION

62-yr-old man presenting with a short history of rectal bleeding associated with change in bowel habits.

PHYSICAL EXAM

INSPECTION: No abnormalities seen.

DIGITAL EXAM: No lesions palpable.

SIGMOIDOSCOPY: Nearly circumferential lesion 9 cm from the anal verge. The lesion has some villous features but the base is hard (Fig. 8.23).

TREATMENT: Low anterior resection with stapled anastomosis.

PATHOLOGY: Well-differentiated colonic adenocarcinoma infiltrating the muscularis propria but not into the perirectal fat (Fig. 8.24). There is no evidence of lymph node metastasis.

FOLLOW-UP: Patient is well 2 yr after surgery.

ENDORECTAL SONOGRAPHY

The tumor is located in the right posterolateral aspect of the recum 9 cm from the anal verge (Fig. 8.25). The lesion encompasses two-thirds of the rectal circumference and is 1.5 cm at its maximal depth (Fig. 8.26). The hyperechoic layer corresponding to the submucosa is destroyed and the hypoechoic layer which represents the muscularis propria is thickened consistent with tumor invasion. The hyperechoic layer that corresponds to the perirectal fat interface is irregular in some areas and these findings usually represent focal tumor invasion. In this case no invasion of the perirectal fat was found on microscopic examination. Although edema may mimic tumor invasion, it is also possible that a small area of focal invasion may have been overlooked. Several small lymph nodes are present in other sections which show fine granularity and have a low probability of having tumor metastasis. The sonographic findings are representative of a Dukes B2 tumor.

pT2

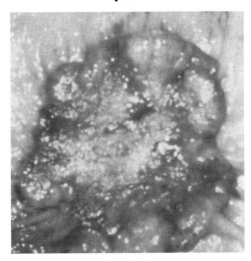

Fig. 8.27

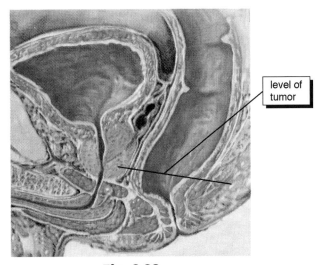

level of
tumor

Fig. 8.28

uT3

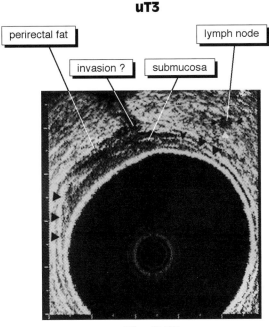

Fig. 8.29

CLINICAL PRESENTATION
75-yr-old man with prostatic cancer presenting with a recent history of rectal bleeding.

PHYSICAL EXAM

INSPECTION: No abnormalities seen.

DIGITAL EXAM: Hard lesion with central ulceration palpable anteriorly at fingertip. The lesion appears mobile (Fig. 8.27).

SIGMOIDOSCOPY: Tumor located 7 cm from the anal verge in the right anterolateral rectal wall (Fig. 8.28). The lesion occupies one-third of the rectal circumference and has friable borders and central ulceration.

TREATMENT: Low anterior resection with stapled anastomosis.

PATHOLOGY: Moderately differentiated adenocarcinoma with deep muscular invasion. No lymph node metastasis seen.

FOLLOW-UP: This patient is free of symptoms 4 yr after surgery but there is a gradual increase in CEA. There is no evidence of recurrence on sigmoidoscopy.

ENDORECTAL SONOGRAPHY
The tumor is located 7 cm from the anal verge and occupies the anterior rectal wall (Fig. 8.29). It is 4 cm in diameter and 1.2 cm in thickness. The surrounding tissues show edema and fibrosis consistent with previous radiotherapy. The hyperechoic layer corresponding to the submucosa is destroyed consistent with tumor invasion. The hypoechoic layer that represents the muscularis propria is thickened which also represents tumor invasion. The hyperechoic layer corresponding to the perirectal fat interface is mostly intact except in one area in the central portion of the tumor where it appears to be infiltrated by tumor. This finding was not confirmed on histologic exam although the tumor invaded deeply into the muscularis propria. One small 0.3 cm lymph node is visible adjacent to the tumor which has a low probability of containing tumor metastasis. The sonographic findings correspond to those of a Dukes B2 lesion with focal invasion of the perirectal fat.

Chapter 9

Perirectal Fat Invasion

Perirectal Fat Invasion

Perirectal fat invasion is diagnosed sonographically by the presence of irregularity of the outer hyperechoic layer which corresponds to the perirectal fat interface. These findings should be associated with disruption of the hyperechoic layer corresponding to the submucosa and thickening of the hypoechoic layer representing the muscularis propria. In some cases, especially when there is narrowing of the lumen and angulation, it may be difficult or impossible to advance the probe proximal to the tumor. Under these circumstances the study may be incomplete and the presence of enlarged lymph nodes may not be ascertained with accuracy since nodes are often located proximal to the tumor.

pT3

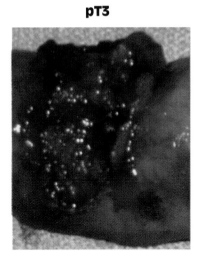

Fig. 9.1

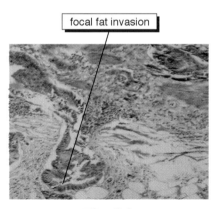

focal fat invasion

Fig. 9.2

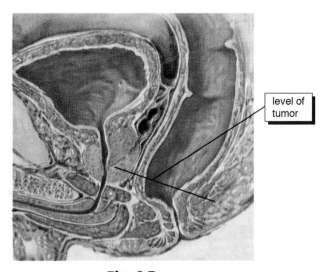

level of tumor

Fig. 9.3

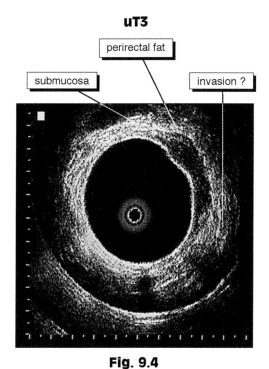

Fig. 9.4

CLINICAL PRESENTATION

66-yr-old man with a 6-month history of rectal bleeding and some narrowing of the stools.

PHYSICAL EXAM

INSPECTION: No external lesions seen.
DIGITAL EXAM: Large, ulcerated, indurated lesion palpable at tip of finger (Fig. 9.1).
SIGMOIDOSCOPY: Polypoid ulcerated lesion located 7 to 8 cm from the anal verge (Fig. 9.3).
TREATMENT: Low anterior resection with everted double-stapled coloanal anastomosis.
PATHOLOGY: Moderately differentiated adenocarcinoma with mucinous features. The tumor invades the entire colonic wall to the perirectal fat (Fig. 9.2). Lymph nodes are free of tumor.
FOLLOW-UP: Patient received chemoradiation following surgery. He is well 3 yr later.

ENDORECTAL SONOGRAPHY

Rectal cancer located 7 cm from the anal verge occupying about 40% of the rectal circumference along the left lateral rectal wall (Fig. 9.4). The lesion is 1.5 cm in maximum depth and 3.5 cm in diameter. The hyperechoic layer corresponding to the submucosa is interrupted and the hypoechoic layer representing the muscularis propria is thickened consistent with tumor invasion. The hyperechoic layer corresponding to the perirectal fat interface is mostly intact although some irregularity is present in some of the sections which represent focal tumor invasion. There are no visible lymph nodes in this study. These findings most likely correspond to those of an early Dukes B2 lesion with focal perirectal fat invasion.

pT3

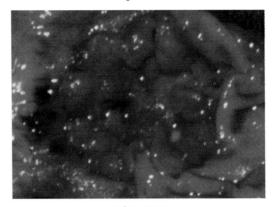

Fig. 9.5

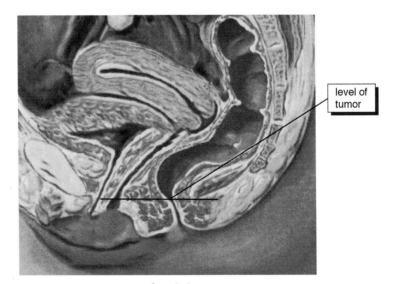

level of
tumor

Fig. 9.6

uT3

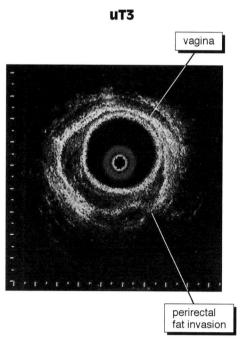

vagina

perirectal
fat invasion

Fig. 9.7

CLINICAL PRESENTATION

79-yr-old woman found to have a rectal cancer on workup for rectal bleeding.

PHYSICAL EXAM

INSPECTION: No external lesions seen.

DIGITAL EXAM: Movable, fungating distal rectal tumor located posteriorly and in the right lateral rectal wall. The lesion occupies at least half of the rectal circumference (Fig. 9.5).

SIGMOIDOSCOPY: Large ulcerated rectal cancer starting just above the dentate line and extending proximally to 9 cm from the anal verge (Fig. 9.6).

TREATMENT: Abdominoperineal resection.

PATHOLOGY: Moderate to poorly differentiated adenocarcinoma with focal colloid features. The tumor extends into the periocolonic fat. Lymph nodes are negative for tumor.

FOLLOW-UP: This patient received postoperative chemoradiation and is free of disease at 3 yr.

ENDORECTAL SONOGRAPHY

Large tumor located at the level of the distal rectum along the posterior and right lateral rectal wall (Fig. 9.7). The lesion occupies nearly 75% of the rectal circumference and distally appears to invade the internal sphincter muscle. The tumor is 1 cm in thickness and 4.5 cm in greatest diameter. Due to its distal location, the submucosal layer is not well seen. The hypoechoic layer corresponding to the muscularis propria is markedly thickened consistent with tumor invasion. The hyperechoic layer representing the perirectal fat interface is irregular, representing focal tumor invasion. There is minimal tumor invasion anteriorly and the posterior vaginal wall appears intact. There are no visible lymph nodes. These findings correspond to those of a Dukes B2 lesion.

pT3

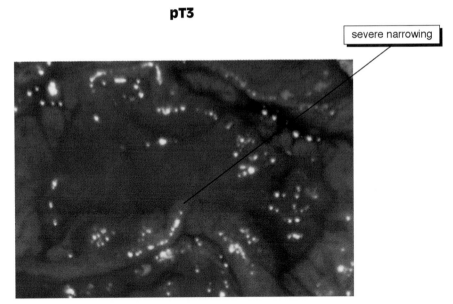

Fig. 9.8

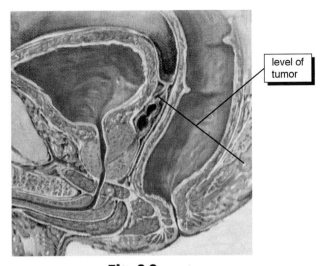

Fig. 9.9

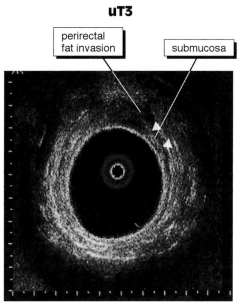

Fig. 9.10

CLINICAL PRESENTATION

64-yr-old man with a 1-yr history of bright red rectal bleeding. Patient also has pain on defecation and stools are pencil thin. He has lost 10 lb in recent months.

PHYSICAL EXAM

INSPECTION: No lesions seen.
DIGITAL EXAM: Tumor not palpable on digital exam.
SIGMOIDOSCOPY: Fixed circumferential lesion 12 to 13 cm from the anal verge (Fig. 9.9). The lumen is severely narrowed and does not allow passage of the rigid sigmoidoscope (Fig. 9.8).
TREATMENT: Anterior resection with everted double-stapled coloanal anastomosis.
PATHOLOGY: Moderately differentiated adenocarcinoma invading the muscularis propria with superficial invasion of the perirectal soft tissue. Lymph nodes are negative for tumor.
FOLLOW-UP: Patient received preoperative radiation and postoperative chemotherapy. He is well 3 yr later.

ENDORECTAL SONOGRAPHY

The endorectal sonography probe could not be inserted past the tumor due to severe narrowing of the lumen. With the probe located at the level of the distal portion of the tumor, the anterior portion was visualized (Fig. 9.10). The hyperechoic layer corresponding to the submucosa is interrupted and the hypoechoic layer representing the muscularis propria is thickened showing tumor invasion. The hyperechoic layer corresponding to the perirectal fat interface is destroyed anteriorly representing tumor invasion into the perirectal fat. There are no lymph nodes seen below the tumor. The area proximal to the tumor could not be evaluated since the probe could not be advanced beyond the tumor. These findings correspond to a Dukes B2 lesion.

pT3

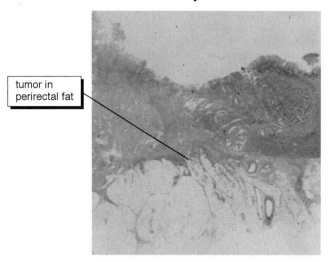

tumor in
perirectal fat

Fig. 9.11

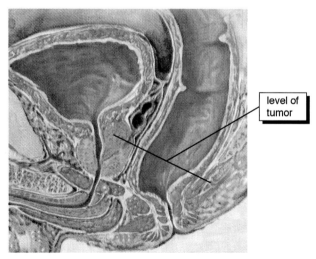

level of
tumor

Fig. 9.12

uT3

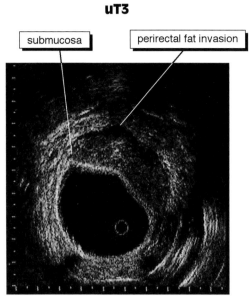

submucosa   perirectal fat invasion

Fig. 9.13

CLINICAL PRESENTATION

42-yr-old patient presenting with 25 lb weight loss, decreased caliber, and guaiac positive stools.

PHYSICAL EXAM

INSPECTION: No lesions seen.

DIGITAL EXAM: Bulky, hard tumor palpable posteriorly.

SIGMOIDOSCOPY: Large polypoid tumor seen 9 cm from the anal verge occupying the left anterolateral circumference of the rectum (Fig. 9.12).

TREATMENT: Low anterior resection with double-stapled coloanal anastomosis.

PATHOLOGY: Moderately differentiated colonic adenocarcinoma infiltrating into the perirectal fat (Fig. 9.11). Lymph nodes are negative for tumor.

FOLLOW-UP: This patient received postoperative chemoradiation and is well 3 yr later.

ENDORECTAL SONOGRAPHY

Bulky tumor is present 9 cm from the anal verge occupying nearly 50% of the rectal circumference (Fig. 9.13). The tumor extends for a depth of 1.5 cm, is 5 cm in diameter, and appears to penetrate the perirectal fat. Deep penetration is represented by destruction of the hyperechoic layer corresponding to the submucosa, marked thickening of the hypoechoic muscularis propria, and irregularity of the hyperechoic perirectal fat interface. Two small lymph nodes 0.3 cm in diameter are visible in one of the sections. Because of their small size, these nodes have a low probability of containing metastatic cancer. The findings correspond to those of a Dukes B2 lesion.

pT3

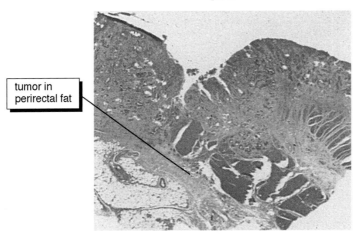

tumor in
perirectal fat

Fig. 9.14

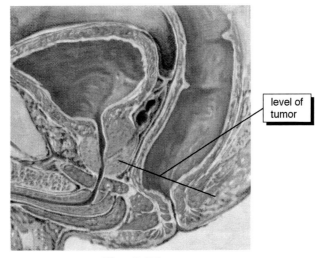

level of
tumor

Fig. 9.15

uT3

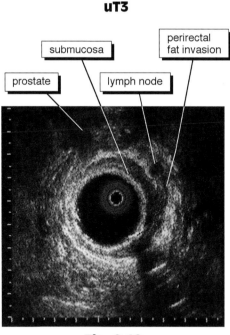

prostate

submucosa

lymph node

perirectal
fat invasion

Fig. 9.16

CLINICAL PRESENTATION

78-yr-old man presenting with a 6-month history of rectal bleeding.

PHYSICAL EXAM

INSPECTION: No lesions seen.

DIGITAL EXAM: Ulcerated lesion palpable on left lateral rectal wall.

SIGMOIDOSCOPY: Ulcerated tumor starting at dentate line, located on the left lateral rectal wall and extending for a distance of 6 cm (Fig. 9.15).

TREATMENT: Abdominoperineal resection.

PATHOLOGY: Moderately differentiated adenocarcinoma infiltrating into the perirectal fat (Fig. 9.14). Lymph nodes are negative for tumor.

FOLLOW-UP: Patient is well 3 yr later.

ENDORECTAL SONOGRAPHY

Rectal cancer located on the left lateral rectal wall occupying about 60% of the rectal circumference (Fig. 9.16). The tumor is 1.3 cm in depth and 5 cm in diameter. The hyperechoic line corresponding to the submucosa is destroyed and the hypoechoic line representing the muscularis propria is thickened consistent with tumor invasion. The hyperechoic layer representing the perirectal fat interface shows irregularity characteristic of tumor invasion. Several small lymph nodes are present which have a low to moderate probability of containing metastatic disease. These findings are consistent with a deeply invading cancer with a low probability of nodal metastasis. This sonogram represents a Dukes B2 lesion.

pT3

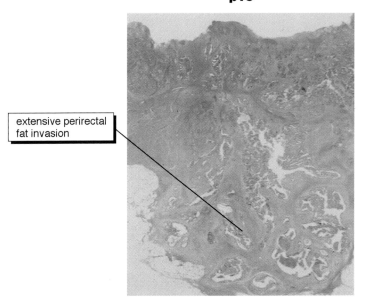

extensive perirectal
fat invasion

Fig. 9.17

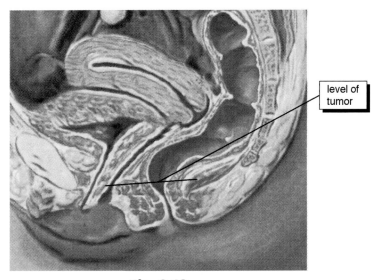

level of
tumor

Fig. 9.18

uT3

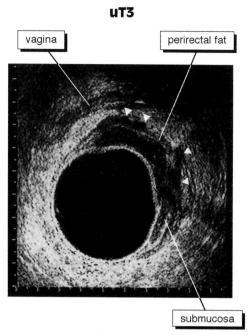

vagina | perirectal fat

submucosa

Fig. 9.19

CLINICAL PRESENTATION

56-yr-old woman presenting with a 1-yr history of rectal bleeding and more recently having pencil thin stools.

PHYSICAL EXAM

INSPECTION: External hemorrhoids.

DIGITAL EXAM: Hard ulcerated mass anteriorly.

SIGMOIDOSCOPY: Anterior ulcerated mass located 5 cm from the anal verge (Fig. 9.18).

TREATMENT: Low anterior resection with everted double-stapled coloanal anastomosis.

PATHOLOGY: Moderately differentiated adenocarcinoma infiltrating the perirectal fat (Fig. 9.17). Lymph nodes are free of tumor.

FOLLOW-UP: Patient refused chemoradiation after surgery. She developed a recurrence at the anastomosis which required an abdominoperineal resection 6 months later.

ENDORECTAL SONOGRAPHY

Large tumor occupying half the rectal circumference on the left anterolateral side and located 5 cm from the anal verge (Fig. 9.19). The tumor is nearly 2 cm in depth and 6 cm in diameter. The hyperechoic line corresponding to the submucosa is destroyed and the hypoechoic layer representing the muscularis propria is markedly thickened consistent with tumor invasion. The hyperechoic layer representing the perirectal fat interface is irregular consistent with extensive tumor invasion. There are no visible lymph nodes. These findings are seen with a deeply infiltrating Dukes B2 tumor.

Chapter 10

Extensive Local Invasion

Extensive Local Invasion

This section shows examples of locally advanced tumors with deep invasion beyond the bowel wall. These features are well seen on endorectal sonography. Some of these patients also had distant spread, usually liver metastasis. We have treated patients with advanced local disease with preoperative chemoradiation followed by abdominoperineal resection. Some patients with residual tumor in the pelvis had intraoperative brachytherapy but the results have not been very encouraging.

pT4

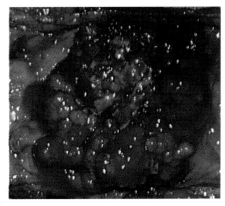

Fig. 10.1

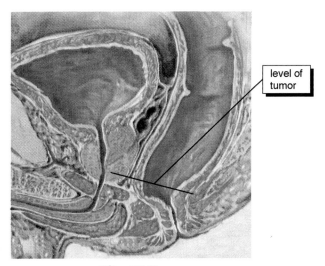

level of tumor

Fig. 10.2

uT4

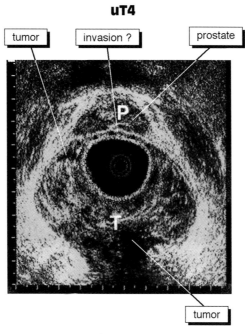

tumor | invasion ? | prostate

tumor

Fig. 10.3

CLINICAL PRESENTATION

57-yr-old man with a longstanding history of rectal bleeding and recent onset of tenesmus.

PHYSICAL EXAM

INSPECTION: No external lesions seen.

DIGITAL EXAM: Circumferential exophytic mass with a hard base fixed posteriorly to the sacrum (Fig. 10.1).

SIGMOIDOSCOPY: Large circumferential rectal cancer arising just above the dentate line (Fig. 10.2).

TREATMENT: Palliative abdominoperineal resection.

PATHOLOGY: Well-differentiated adenocarcinoma with colloid features infiltrating into the perirectal fat. Lymph nodes are free of tumor.

FOLLOW-UP: Patient was treated with chemoradiation after surgery and was subsequently lost to follow-up.

ENDORECTAL SONOGRAPHY

Large, fungating rectal cancer extending from just above the anal verge for a distance of 10 cm (Fig. 10.3). The distal portion is a circumferential deeply ulcerated cancer invading through the rectal wall into the perirectal fat and extending to the pelvic side wall. The normal sonographic layers are no longer visible due to extensive tumor invasion. The tumor is at least 3 cm in depth and appears to invade the prostatic capsule anteriorly. There are no visible lymph nodes. These findings correspond to those seen with a lesion invading the pelvic side wall.

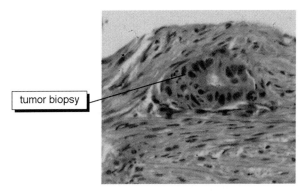

Fig. 10.4

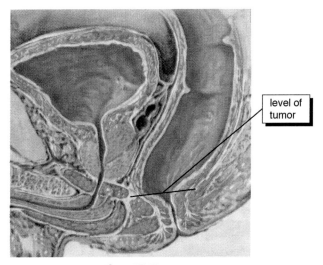

Fig. 10.5

uT4

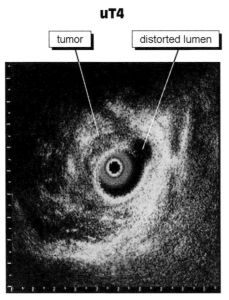

tumor   distorted lumen

Fig. 10.6

CLINICAL PRESENTATION
49-yr-old man presenting with rectal bleeding, weight loss, and tenesmus.

PHYSICAL EXAM

INSPECTION: No lesions seen.

DIGITAL EXAM: Large fixed hard mass present just above the anal verge with severe narrowing and distortion of the lumen (Fig. 10.5).

SIGMOIDOSCOPY: Could not be performed due to narrowing and distortion caused by the tumor.

TREATMENT: Chemoradiation.

PATHOLOGY: Moderately differentiated rectal adenocarcinoma on biopsy (Fig. 10.4).

FOLLOW-UP: Patient refused abdominoperineal resection. He underwent chemoradiation and is alive 1 yr later with extensive pelvic tumor.

ENDORECTAL SONOGRAPHY
Only the distal portion of the tumor could be evaluated due to narrowing and distortion of the rectal lumen (Fig. 10.6). A large cancer is seen occupying nearly the entire rectal circumference with severe distortion of the lumen. The tumor is most extensive in the right rectal wall where it is up to 5 cm in thickness and extends to the pelvic side wall. The anterior and posterior components are similar and the tumor is less extensive in the left lateral rectal wall. Due to the extensive nature of the tumor and inability to place the probe past the tumor, the presence of enlarged lymph nodes could not be evaluated.

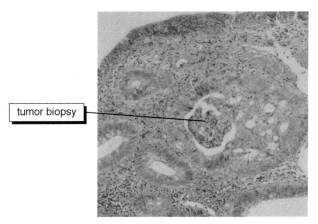

Fig. 10.7

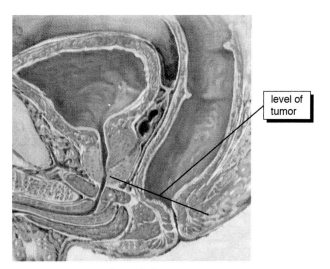

Fig. 10.8

uT4

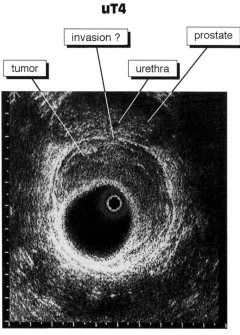

Fig. 10.9

CLINICAL PRESENTATION

59-yr-old man presenting with rectal bleeding, narrow stools and tenesmus.

PHYSICAL EXAM

INSPECTION: No external lesions seen.

DIGITAL EXAM: Hard, fixed, large tumor palpable anteriorly occupying nearly two-thirds of the rectal circumference.

SIGMOIDOSCOPY: Nearly circumferential tumor starting just above the dentate line (Fig. 10.8).

TREATMENT: Chemoradiation.

PATHOLOGY: Moderately well-differentiated adenocarcinoma with some villous features on biopsy (Fig. 10.7).

FOLLOW-UP: A CAT scan showed multiple liver metastasis. The patient refused a palliative abdominoperineal resection.

ENDORECTAL SONOGRAPHY

Extensive anterior rectal cancer located at the level of the prostate with possible capsular invasion (Fig. 10.9). The tumor is about 2 cm in greatest depth and 6 cm in diameter. The sonographic layers of the rectal wall are completely disrupted by the tumor. There are no visible lymph nodes. These findings correspond to those of an advanced deeply invasive rectal cancer extending through the bowel wall with possible invasion of the prostatic capsule. Since the patient was found to also have liver metastasis, the tumor stage is Dukes D.

Chapter 11
Lymph Node Metastasis

Lymph Node Metastasis

Sonographic evaluation of lymph node metastasis is somewhat less accurate than depth of invasion. Normal perirectal nodes are not usually seen on endorectal sonography. Enlarged lymph nodes may be hyperplastic or contain metastatic disease. The most reliable criteria for nodal metastasis is the size of the lymph node. Lymph nodes greater than 0.5 cm in diameter have a higher probability of containing metastasis when compared to smaller nodes. Another criterion that helps in the evaluation is the presence of hypoechoic areas and irregular borders which are also more likely to represent metastasis.

pT3,N0

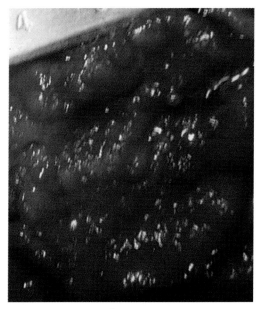

Fig. 11.1

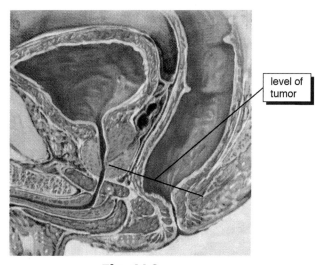

level of
tumor

Fig. 11.2

uT3,N1

| prostate | perirectal fat | lymph node |

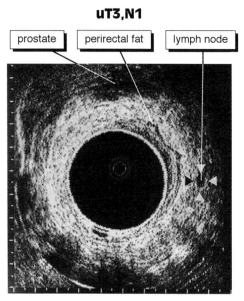

Fig. 11.3

CLINICAL PRESENTATION

83-yr-old man presenting with rectal bleeding.

PHYSICAL EXAM

INSPECTION: No lesions seen.

DIGITAL EXAM: Hard lesion occupying half of the circumference located in the anterior and left lateral rectal wall (Fig. 11.1).

SIGMOIDOSCOPY: Tumor located 5 cm from the anal verge, with some villous features with indurated central portion (Fig. 11.2).

TREATMENT: Abdominoperineal resection.

PATHOLOGY: Poorly differentiated rectal adenocarcinoma extending into the perirectal fat. Regional lymph nodes are free of tumor.

FOLLOW-UP: Patient is well 4 yr after surgery.

ENDORECTAL SONOGRAPHY

Tumor 4 cm in diameter located in the left anterolateral rectal wall 5 cm from the anal verge (Fig. 11.3). The lesion is 0.7 cm in greatest depth. The hyperechoic layer corresponding to the submucosa is broken and the hypoechoic layer representing the muscularis propria is thickened consistent with tumor invasion. The hyperechoic layer corresponding to the perirectal fat interface is irregular indicating invasion of the perirectal fat. One lymph node is visible adjacent to the tumor. This node is 0.5 cm in diameter, elliptical in outline, and hypoechoic. These findings correspond to a deeply infiltrating cancer with a moderate probability of nodal metastasis. This tumor is sonographically a Dukes C2 lesion. This is an example of a hyperplastic lymph node appearing as a possible nodal metastasis.

pT2,N1

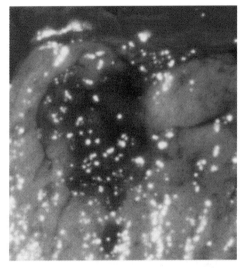

Fig. 11.4

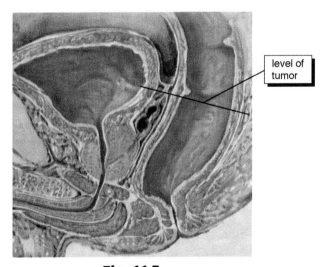

level of
tumor

Fig. 11.5

uT2,N1

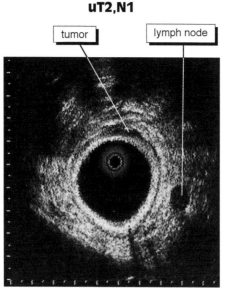

tumor | lymph node

Fig. 11.6

CLINICAL PRESENTATION

63-yr-old man found to have guaiac positive stools on physical exam.

PHYSCIAL EXAM

INSPECTION: No lesions seen.

DIGITAL EXAM: No palpable lesions.

SIGMOIDOSCOPY: 3-cm tumor located 11 cm from the anal verge (Fig. 11.4).

TREATMENT: Low anterior resection with stapled distal rectal anastomosis.

PATHOLOGY: Poorly differentiated adenocarcinoma invading the muscularis propria. Two lymph nodes contain metastatic carcinoma.

FOLLOW-UP: This patient received chemoradiation following surgery. He is well 2 yr postoperatively.

ENDORECTAL SONOGRAPHY

Rectal tumor located 11 cm from the anal verge (Fig. 11.5). The lesion is 2.5 cm in diameter and 0.5 cm in depth (Fig. 11.6). The hyperechoic layer corresponding to the submucosal layer is disrupted and the hypoechoic layer representing the muscularis is thickened consistent with tumor invasion. The hyperechoic line which represents the perirectal fat interface is intact. Adjacent to the tumor is a large lymph node which is 0.8 cm in diameter and hypoechoic. Adjacent to it but not seen in this section is another node 0.6 cm in diameter of similar echogenicity. These findings correspond to a superficially invasive lesion extending to the muscularis propria with lymph node metastasis. This is a Dukes C1 lesion.

pT2,N1

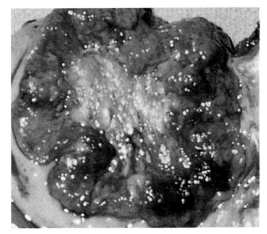

Fig. 11.7

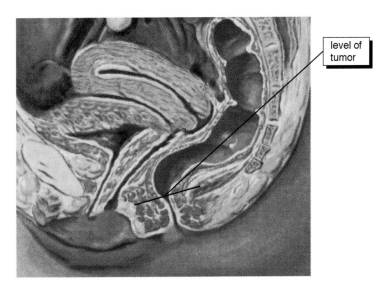

level of
tumor

Fig. 11.8

uT2,N1

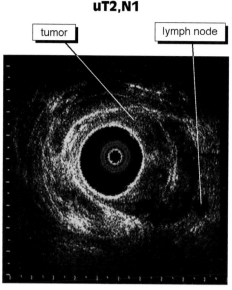

Fig. 11.9

CLINICAL PRESENTATION

64-yr-old woman presenting with rectal bleeding and weight loss.

PHYSCIAL EXAM

INSPECTION: No external lesions seen.

DIGITAL EXAM: Large nearly circumferential lesion with villous features and central ulceration (Fig. 11.7).

SIGMOIDOSCOPY: Circumferential lesion starting at dentate line (Fig. 11.8). Some areas show a soft villous component but the central area is hard and ulcerated.

TREATMENT: Abdominoperineal resection.

PATHOLOGY: Moderately differentiated adenocarcimona infiltrating into the muscularis propria. Three lymph nodes are positive for metastatic carcinoma.

FOLLOW-UP: Intraoperative biopsy of a small liver nodule not seen on preoperative computerized axial tomography (CAT) scan showed metastatic carcinoma.

ENDORECTAL SONOGRAPHY

Rectal lesion most prominent in the left lateral rectal wall, nearly circumferential except for a small free portion in the right lateral rectal wall (Fig. 11.9). The hyperechoic layer representing the submucosa is interrupted and the hypoechoic layer corresponding to the muscularis is markedly thickened consistent with tumor invasion. The tumor is 3 cm in greatest thickness and nearly 7 cm in diameter. The hyperechoic layer corresponding to the perirectal fat interface is intact. Three lymph nodes are present varying in size from 0.6 to 1 cm in diameter. These nodes are hypoechoic and have irregular borders. Their size, lack of echogenicity, and irregular outline correlate with a high probability of metastatic disease. These findings are consistent with a Dukes C1 lesion although the presence of a liver metastasis changes it to a Dukes D lesion.

pT3,N1
Post RT

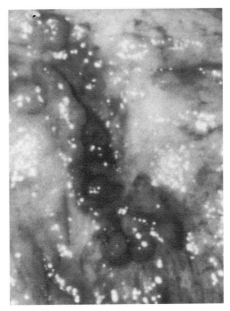

Fig. 11.10

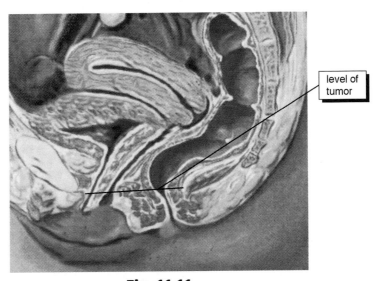

level of
tumor

Fig. 11.11

uT3,N1
Pre RT

tumor   lymph node

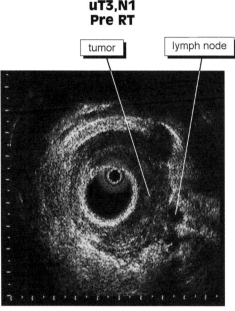

Fig. 11.12

CLINICAL PRESENTATION

56-yr-old woman presenting with a 2-month history of rectal bleeding associated with 6 lb weight loss.

PHYSICAL EXAM

INSPECTION: No abnormalities seen.

DIGITAL EXAM: Nearly circumferential lesion in the distal rectum.

SIGMOIDOSCOPY: Fungating lesion 5 cm from the anal verge occupying most of the rectal circumference (Fig. 11.11).

TREATMENT: Abdominoperineal resection.

PATHOLOGY: Adenocarcinoma with colloid features invading the perirectal fat. Two lymph nodes contain metastatic carcinoma.

FOLLOW-UP: This patient received preoperative chemoradiation which resulted in significant tumor regression (Fig. 11.10).

ENDORECTAL SONOGRAPHY

Large, nearly circumferential rectal cancer located mostly along the left lateral rectal wall (Fig. 11.12). The tumor is about 1.5 cm in depth. There is destruction of the hyperechoic line corresponding to the submucosa and marked thickening of the hypoechoic layer representing the muscularis consistent with tumor invasion. The hyperechoic layer corresponding to the perirectal fat interface is also destroyed. Several lymph nodes ranging in size from 0.5 to 1 cm in diameter are seen. Some are hypoechoic with irregular borders with a high probability of metastatic disease. These findings correspond to those of a Dukes C2 lesion.

**pT3,N1
Post RT**

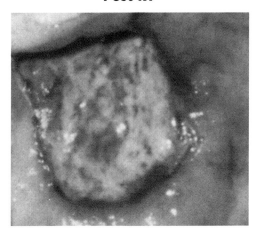

Fig. 11.13

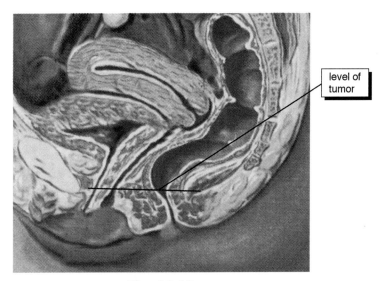

level of
tumor

Fig. 11.14

uT3,N1
Pre RT

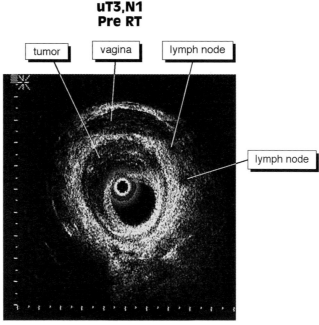

Fig. 11.15

CLINICAL PRESENTATION

31-yr-old woman presenting with an advanced rectal cancer.

PHYSICAL EXAM

INSPECTION: No abnormalities seen.

DIGITIAL EXAM: Hard tumor with narrow residual lumen located just above the anal verge.

SIGMOIDOSCOPY: Large, friable, nearly circumferential rectal cancer starting at dentate line (Fig. 11.14).

TREATMENT: Abdominoperineal resection.

PATHOLOGY: Colloid carcinoma invading the perirectal fat. Tumor is present in the rectovaginal septum. Five lymph nodes contain metastatic carcinoma.

FOLLOW-UP: This patient underwent chemoradiation prior to surgery with partial regression of the tumor (Fig. 11.13).

ENDORECTAL SONOGRAPHY

Extensive deeply infiltrating rectal cancer 5 cm from the anal verge (Fig. 11.15). The tumor occupies over two-thirds of the rectal circumference and in some areas the thickness is 2 cm. There is destruction of the hyperechoic layer corresponding to the submucosa and severe thickening of the hypoechoic layer representing the muscularis propria. The hyperechoic layer corresponding to the perirectal fat interface is irregular consistent with tumor invasion. The posterior vaginal wall is very close to the tumor. Multiple lymph nodes ranging from 0.5 to 1 cm in diameter are visible. They are hypoechoic and have a high probability of containing metastatic disease. These findings correspond to those of a Dukes C2 tumor.

pT3,N1

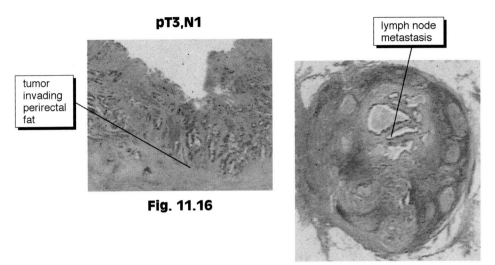

tumor invading perirectal fat

lymph node metastasis

Fig. 11.16

Fig. 11.17

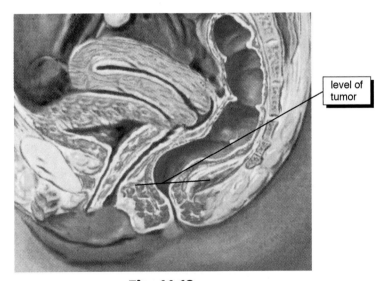

level of tumor

Fig. 11.18

uT3,N1

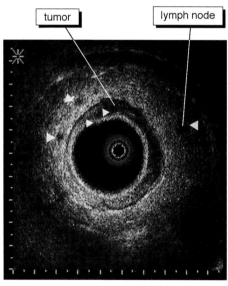

Fig. 11.19

CLINICAL PRESENTATION

77-yr-old woman presenting with urgency and increased frequency of bowel movements.

PHYSICAL EXAM

INSPECTION: No external abnormalities seen.

DIGITAL EXAM: Movable circumferential tumor palpable at tip of finger.

SIGMOIDOSCOPY: Nearly circumferential tumor 7 cm from the anal verge (Fig. 11.18).

TREATMENT: Low anterior resection with everted double-stapled coloanal anastomosis.

PATHOLOGY: Infiltrating moderately differentiated adenocarcinoma. The tumor invades the entire rectal wall to the perirectal fat (Fig. 11.16). Metastatic carcinoma is present in two lymph nodes (Fig. 11.17).

FOLLOW-UP: Patient received adjuvant chemoradiotherapy postoperatively.

ENDORECTAL SONOGRAPHY

Rectal tumor 7 cm from the anal verge occupying three-quarters of the rectal circumference mostly on the left, anterior and posterior rectal walls (Fig. 11.19). The tumor is 1 cm in depth. The hyperechoic layer corresponding to the submucosa is destroyed and the hypoechoic layer representing the muscularis is thickened consistent with tumor invasion. The hyperechoic layer corresponding to the perirectal fat interface is irregular and therefore invaded by tumor. Three small lymph nodes less than 0.5 cm in diameter are visible in the right lateral rectal wall and a larger node 0.8 cm in diameter is seen in the left lateral rectal wall. The larger node is hypoechoic and has irregular borders consistent with tumor metastasis. These findings correspond to those of a Dukes C2 lesion.

pT3,N1

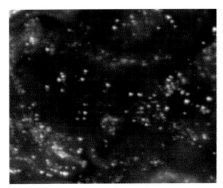

Fig. 11.20

lymph node metastasis

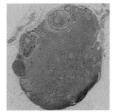

Fig. 11.21

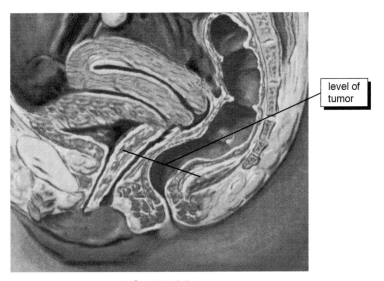

level of tumor

Fig. 11.22

uT3,N0

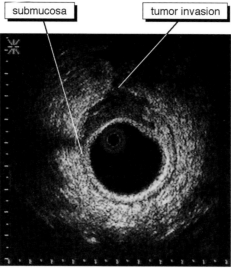

Fig. 11.23

CLINICAL PRESENTATION

67-yr-old woman presenting with 1-yr history of rectal bleeding and recent increase in frequency of bowel movements.

PHYSICAL EXAM

INSPECTION: No abnormalities seen.
DIGITAL EXAM: Circumferential movable lesion palpable at tip of finger (Fig. 11.20).
SIGMOIDOSCOPY: Circumferential tumor located 10 cm from the anal verge (Fig. 11.22).
TREATMENT: Low anterior resection with mucosectomy and hand-sewn coloanal anastomosis.
PATHOLOGY: Well-differentiated colonic adenocarcinoma with transmural invasion and metastasis to one lymph node (Fig. 11.21).
FOLLOW-UP: This patient received adjuvant chemoradiation following surgery. The tumor recurred in the rectum 1.5 yr later requiring abdominoperineal resection.

ENDORECTAL SONOGRAPHY

The ultrasound probe could not be inserted beyond the tumor due to narrowing and angulation of the lumen. The distal portion of the tumor was seen 10 cm from the anal verge occupying the anterior rectal wall (Fig. 11.23). The tumor is 1.5 cm in depth at this level and extends through the hyperechoic submucosa and the hypoechoic muscularis. The hyperechoic layer corresponding to the perirectal fat interface is broken consistent with tumor invasion. There are no visible nodes but since the study is incomplete, the possibility of nodal metastasis cannot be ruled out. These findings correspond to those of a Dukes B2 lesion. The single lymph node with metastatic disease was located proximal to the tumor.

pT3,N1

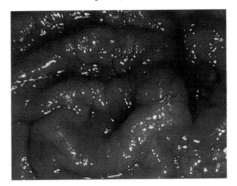

Fig. 11.24

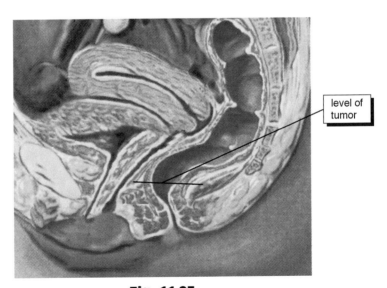

level of
tumor

Fig. 11.25

uT3,N1

lymph node

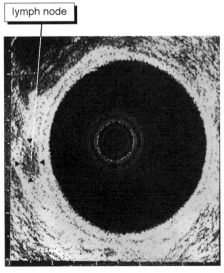

Fig. 11.26

CLINICAL PRESENTATION

41-yr-old woman with a history of rectal bleeding for 6 months associated with some decrease in the caliber of the stools.

PHYSICAL EXAM

INSPECTION: No external lesions seen.

DIGITAL EXAM: Tumor palpable at tip of finger. Lesion is movable and has rasied edges with central ulceration (Fig. 11.24).

SIGMOIDOSCOPY: Ulcerated lesion located 6 cm from the anal verge about 3 × 2 cm in diameter with central ulceration (Fig. 11.25).

TREATMENT: Low anterior resection with everted stapled coloanal anastomosis.

PATHOLOGY: Moderately differentiated adenocarcinoma extending into the pericolonic fat. One lymph node contains metastatic carcinoma.

FOLLOW-UP: This patient received chemoradiation following surgery. She is well 5 yr later.

ENDORECTAL SONOGRAPHY

Tumor 3 cm in diameter located in the anterior rectal wall 6 cm from the anal verge (not shown). The tumor is about 1 cm in depth and the hyperechoic line representing the submucosa is disrupted. The hypoechoic layer corresponding to the rectal muscularis is thickened and the hyperechoic line at the perirectal fat interface is disrupted consistent with deep tumor invasion. A large lymph node about 0.8 cm in diameter is seen proximal to the tumor near the right lateral rectal wall (Fig. 11.26). This lymph node is hypoechoic and has an irregular outline consistent with tumor metastasis. These findings correspond to those of a Dukes C2 lesion.

pT2,N1

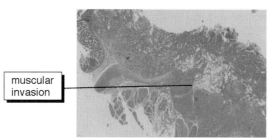

Fig. 11.27

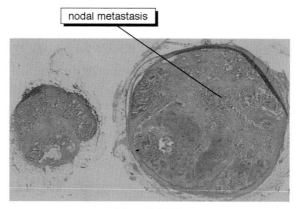

Fig. 11.28

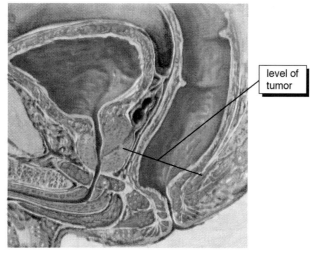

Fig. 11.29

uT2,N1

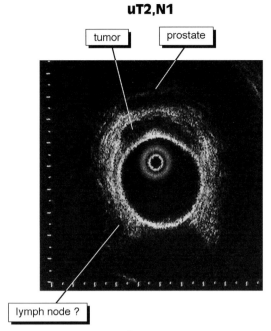

Fig. 11.30

CLINICAL PRESENTATION

48-yr-old man presenting with a 1-yr history of rectal bleeding.

PHYSICAL EXAM

INSPECTION: No external lesions seen.

DIGITAL EXAM: Movable anterior tumor palpable at tip of finger, occupying one-half of the rectal circumference.

SIGMOIDOSCOPY: Rectal cancer at 6 cm from the anal verge, about 4 cm in diameter (Fig. 11.29).

TREATMENT: Low anterior resection with mucosectomy and hand-sewn coloanal anastomosis.

PATHOLOGY: Moderately differentiated adenocarcinoma invading the muscularis propria. (Fig. 11.27) Two adjacent lymph nodes contain metastatic carcinoma (Fig. 11.28).

FOLLOW-UP: This patient had chemoradiation following surgery and is well 3 yr later.

ENDORECTAL SONOGRAPHY

Anterior rectal cancer approximately 3.5 cm in diameter located 6 cm from the anal verge. (Fig. 11.30) The tumor is 0.8 cm in thickness and the hyperechoic layer corresponding to the submucosa is disrupted. The hypoechoic layer representing the muscularis is thickened consistent with tumor invasion. The outer hyperechoic layer representing the perirectal fat interface is intact. There are no clearly visible lymph nodes either adjacent or proximal to the tumor although in the right posterolateral area at the level of the tumor is a structure that probably represents a partially seen hypoechoic node. These findings correspond to those of a superficially invasive tumor with a possible metastatic node adjacent to the tumor (Dukes C2).

pT4,N1

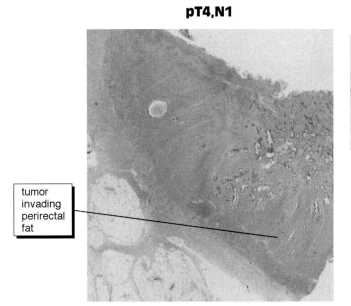

Fig. 11.31

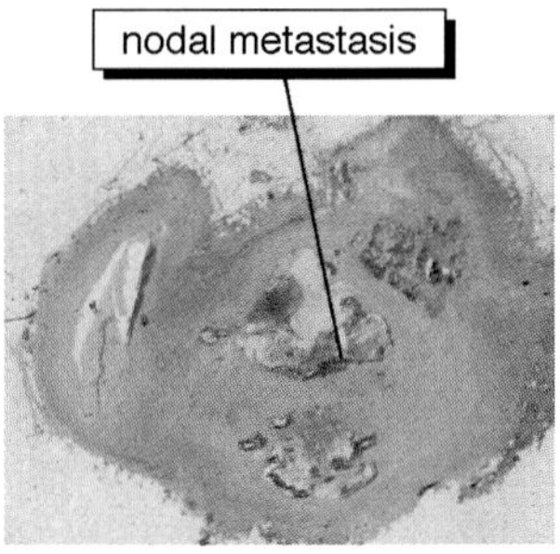

Fig. 11.32

nodal metastasis

tumor invading perirectal fat

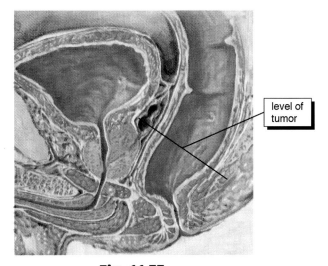

level of tumor

Fig. 11.33

uT3,N1

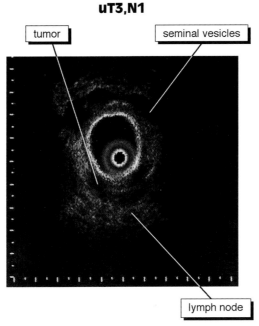

tumor

seminal vesicles

lymph node

Fig. 11.34

CLINICAL PRESENTATION

59-yr-old man who initially refused treatment for rectal cancer and now presents with an advanced tumor which has been treated with chemoradiation.

PHYSICAL EXAM

INSPECTION: No external abnormalities seen.
DIGITAL EXAM: Hard, circumferential tumor palpable at tip of finger (Fig. 11.33).
SIGMOIDOSCOPY: Unable to perform rigid sigmoidoscopy due to marked luminal narrowing.
TREATMENT: Abdominoperineal resection.
PATHOLOGY: Moderate to poorly differentiated adenocarcinoma invading to the right pelvic side wall (Fig. 11.31). One adjacent lymph node contains metastatic carcinoma (Fig. 11.32).
FINDINGS: This patient had residual tumor posteriorly and in the right lateral pelvic wall which was treated with intraoperative brachytherapy.

ENDORECTAL SONOGRAPHY

Due to severe narrowing of the lumen and angulation, the ultrasound probe could only be advanced to the distal margin of the tumor. Deeply invading residual tumor was seen in the posterior rectal wall (Fig. 11.34). This tumor is about 3.5 cm in diameter and 1 cm in depth. The normal layers of the bowel wall are difficult to see due to destruction by the tumor and previous radiation. The hyperechoic submucosal layer is nearly completely destroyed and the hypoechoic muscularis propria is markedly thickened by tumor invasion. The hyperechoic perirectal fat interface is irregular representing tumor invasion. Two round hypoechoic shadows are present posterior to the tumor and represent lymph nodes. One is nearly 1 cm in diameter and the outline is irregular. These findings represent extensive residual disease with full-thickness penetration and nodal metastasis. The sonographic appearance is that of a Dukes C2 tumor.

Index

References in italics denote figures; those followed by "t" denote tables